THIRD

Health Care

A Basic Guide

Cost Management

THIRD EDITION

Health Care

A Basic Guide

Cost Management

► Madelon Lubin Finkel ◄

INTERNATIONAL FOUNDATION OF EMPLOYEE BENEFIT PLANS

The opinions expressed in this book are those of the author.
The International Foundation of Employee Benefit Plans disclaims
responsibility for views expressed and statements made in books
published by the Foundation.

Edited by Judith A. Sankey

Copies of this book may be obtained from:
    Publications Department
    International Foundation of Employee Benefit Plans
    18700 West Bluemound Road
    P.O. Box 69
    Brookfield, Wisconsin 53008-0069
    (414) 786-6710, ext. 8240

Payment must accompany order.
Call (888) 33-IFEBP (888-334-3327) for price information.

Published in 1996 by the International Foundation of Employee Benefit Plans, Inc.
©1996 International Foundation of Employee Benefit Plans, Inc.
All rights reserved.
Library of Congress Catalog Card Number: 96-76749
ISBN 0-89154-498-4
Printed in the United States of America

1M-796

Dedication

To my wonderful daughter, Rebecca Finkel

Table of Contents

Acknowledgments

Sincere thanks and appreciation are extended to Clarissa Crabtree for her excellent administrative and editing skills. Without her amazing computer know-how, the text would be less interesting. Her contribution is much appreciated.

Thanks are also extended to Lena Casimir, a premedical student, who spent a summer researching information on substance abuse in the United States. Much of what Lena prepared was incorporated into the chapter on substance abuse.

About the Author

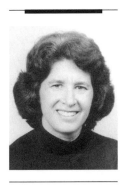

M adelon Lubin Finkel is a nationwide expert on health care issues. She holds the rank of professor of clinical public health at Cornell University Medical College, where she has been part of the faculty for almost 20 years. Dr. Finkel is also principal and owner of MLF Management (formerly Second Opinion Consultants, Inc.), a nationwide health care organization dedicated to health care cost management. Dr. Finkel earned her B.A. at University College, New York University and her M.P.A. and Ph.D. also at New York University. She has also served as consultant to numerous corporations and trust funds in the area of health care cost management and has written extensively in this area. Her other books include the first and second editions of *Health Care Cost Management—A Basic Guide* and *Retiree Health Care: A Ticking Time Bomb,* all published by the International Foundation of Employee Benefit Plans. Dr. Finkel is a charter member of the Foundation's Academy of Employee Benefit Authors.

Introduction

Health care in the United States is generally acknowledged to be among the best in the world. It is also common knowledge that the United States spends more on health care than any other nation, yet it does not rank in the top ten in infant mortality or life expectancy. Most other health care systems in the developed nations insure virtually all of their citizens, allow them the freedom to select their own doctor, and basically constrain medical expenditures at a level that is politically and economically acceptable. While there are problems inherent in these other health care systems, it is the American system that heads the list in costs per person and per unit service as well as in overall dissatisfaction. Hence, one could conclude that despite vast expenditures for health care, the U.S. system is providing neither universal coverage (note our 40 million-plus uninsured population) nor a higher health status, which other nations enjoy for comparatively less money and greater satisfaction.

The failure to achieve a more disciplined health care system has had serious financial ramifications. Health outlays as a share of total labor compensation (wages, salaries and fringe benefits) have soared and the cost of providing health benefits continues to account for an increasingly greater proportion of employers' benefits expenditures. Benefit costs still represent a substantial portion of total payroll. Not surprisingly, the question of who will pay for increasing health care costs has dominated collective bargaining in the past years.

While there is little disagreement that the system needs to be changed or reformed, the methods of effecting such change often provoke passionate differences of opinion. If one were to poll ten people and elicit their thoughts on how the system should be reformed, it would not be surprising to get ten different opinions. As we approach the 21st century, this author maintains that employers and trust funds can, and should, be key players in reforming the health care delivery system. Primarily because the majority of Americans obtain health coverage through their employer and many retirees receive retiree health benefits from their former employer, the employer's role cannot be ignored. Moreover, for decades, employee health benefits have been financed by employers and, as the costs of these benefits soared, employers realized that they had to take a more proactive role to better manage their health care dollars. Astute benefits professionals certainly recognize that the health care cost problem does little to enable an organization to remain competitive. So, what were employers and unions doing about the situation besides individually implementing cost-containment programs?

The purchasers of care began to search aggressively for options to control their hemorrhaging costs. During the 1980s, for example, most employers adopted health care cost-containment programs designed to reduce unnecessary expenditures and inappropriate utilization as well as to encourage alternatives to costly in-hospital care. The volume and intensity of services had been the driving force behind increasing health care costs. The growth in the sheer number of services (volume) and a shift in physician practice patterns for a given condition or diagnosis (intensity) fueled the system. Increased service use resulted from a greater utilization of tests and procedures and from the substitution of more sophisticated tests for previously used simpler ones, or from a combination thereof. Unfortunately, past efforts of revamping, restructuring and reorganizing did not really address the important issues of cost inflation or lack of coverage. The goal continues to be the design of a more efficient delivery system to promote the appropriate use of health care resources for all.

Events in the health care sector were happening so fast that it was often difficult to figure out what should or could be done. In hindsight, the piecemeal cost-containment efforts were unlikely to reduce the growth of overall health spending significantly. The fragmented, complex payment system and the micromanaged administered system were (and still are) inherently inefficient. Frustrated by the mediocre results of early cost-containment programs, and stymied by the lack of agreement on how health care should be reformed, numerous business coalitions (consortiums of employers) were formed. Business realized that more could be achieved as a collective force rather than by each acting independently. While some coalitions are more sophisticated than others, all are involved in projects monitoring costs and quality of care in their communities. Data are collected, outcomes analyzed, surveys conducted, and education and information disseminated. Additionally, small businesses joined forces to form health purchasing alliances, which are designed to give these businesses access to more affordable health care by pooling small businesses into groups for the purpose of buying health insurance products, thereby gaining price breaks that are typically only available to larger groups. In a voluntary market, it is critical that purchasers are able to negotiate price and quality for the products they receive. In order to succeed, alliances have to offer efficient administration and excellent marketing as well as a choice of plans.

Some of the larger alliances include the Florida Community Health Insurance Purchasing Alliance, which has 12,500 small business members representing 56,000 enrolled workers and their dependents; the Kentucky Alliance Plan Source Health Purchasing Alliance, which is now the largest state purchasing alliance in the nation; and the California state-sponsored alliance (Health Insurance Plan of California) covering over 88,000 enrollees.

While the purchasers of care are actively trying to form a cost-efficient system, other players, too, are reshaping how care is delivered and financed. Developing partnerships for a better integrated health care system appears to be the model of the future, and most health care organizations are forging linkages in an attempt to position themselves in the rapidly changing health care environment. Hospitals are merging with other hospitals and buying physician practices at a furious pace. Pharmaceutical companies are consolidating and joining the managed care free-for-all. Joint ventures increased the size of many organizations, and integrated delivery systems were created. Many different players are organizing to provide administrative and marketing functions. In sum, private market forces are acting on their own to transform the system.

The era of corporatization of health care was ushered in when the most recent politically charged debate about health care reform ended in confusion and failure. Frustrated by the lack of a cohesive national health care policy and by the mediocre results of cost-containment programs, a new, huge bureaucratic system designed to manage care was born. The transformation of the health care landscape was swift and dramatic. Employers flocked to this new, untested system in hopes of finally realizing savings.

In this author's opinion, the Clinton administration's laudable but failed attempt to reform the health care system served to unleash market forces, which had been fostered by the Reagan administration's laissez-faire style, creating an industry which is among the fastest growing segment of the economy. This new industry, whose objectives are to manage utilization and price primarily by controlling the type, level and frequency of treatment by restricting the level of reimbursement for services, flourished and profoundly changed the way health care is delivered and financed. Yet, serious medical, legal and economic questions remain unanswered. In particular, what effect will managed care have on quality of care, physician choice and cost increases?

Fortunately, many of the factors that have driven the demand for medical services and increased health care spending are those which we actually can do something about. Dr. Arnold S. Relman, the former editor of the *New England Journal of Medicine,* has commented that at issue is not really whether we as a society can afford the present health care system, but whether we are smart enough to change the system in a way that will enable us to use dollars we are already spending in a more rational, efficient and effective way. For example, the crushing administrative overhead of the present system adds layers of fat to an already corpulent system. Our unhealthy lifestyles add millions to the costs of care. Technology has revolutionized the way medicine is practiced, but at a huge cost. The belief that life can be endlessly maintained, leading to its prolongation at great cost, is an ethical issue which must be addressed. The alphabet soup of programs and organizations created during the past decade has produced a change in the way medical care is organized and financed; but have costs really been contained, or have they been merely shifted to another party? We may have changed the structure and process, but in so doing we have created a new set of problems, which must be addressed. The table presents an accurate, albeit cynical, depiction of the U.S. system.

How did we get to this point? What will it mean for the consumer? For the provider? How will it affect health care costs? Access to quality of care? The focus of this latest edition of *Health Care Cost Management—A Basic Guide* is to make some sense out of the dynamic changes in the health care system. Each chapter details a specific issue and tries to present options for consideration, highlighting most but by no means all of the issues and topics that should be considered. The book attempts to touch on most of the "hot issues" to at least familiarize the reader with the most up-to-date thinking at this writing. Each chapter could be the focus of its own book. The guide, however, is intended to present an overview. Also, the health care system is fluid and in flux. What may be the norm or current thinking in 1996 may very well be outdated in a few short years.

This guide's premise is that in order to continue to plan effective strategies to contain health care costs, it is necessary to understand how we got ourselves into the predicament we are in, what factors influenced the growth in health care expenditures and what options would be effective to better manage these costs.

Chapter 1 focuses on the policies that helped shape the health care system and how past actions laid the foundation for the cost crisis of the latter half of the 20th century. The social, political and economic forces of the past decades have served to mold and shape the U.S. health care system. A historical discussion focuses on the shift in the loci of power, control and influence away from organized medicine to a market-driven, for-profit bureaucracy more concerned with the bottom line.

Society as a whole bears the costs of health care whether through taxes, insurance premiums or out-of-pocket payments. It is universally believed that resources available to meet the demands of health care are limited (note the Oregon experiment), making cost-effective health practices imperative. Chapter 2 focuses on the costs of health care, including the growth and expenditures, contributing factors to this growth, and the implications for employers and trust funds. It is shown that after years of double-digit inflation and increases in premiums, medical inflation and total health benefit costs per employee are beginning to abate. However, benefit costs still increased three times the rate of general inflation even though medical care price inflation slowed, leading one to conclude that some underlying problems in the financing and delivery of health care remain.

TABLE

Health Care Food Chain

Providers Pass Their
Costs to Patients.

Patients Send Bills to
Insurance Company or
Other Third Party Payers.

Insurance Premiums
Increase for Employers.

Employers Cost Shift
to Employees.

So, who ultimately bears the burden of rising health care costs?

WE ALL DO.

This fact should caution the reader to remain vigilant about cost management. Experience suggests that there are no simple solutions to the cost problem.

The first two chapters are intended to illustrate that the health care delivery system is in flux and its configuration is being shaped by a multitude of forces. It is also maintained that health care costs and their effect on employee benefits are intertwined. Chapter 3 focuses on the growth in employee benefits and the means of providing benefits in a cost-efficient manner. It should be made clear that providing employee benefits is not an incidental cost of doing business. Discussion focuses on the types of benefits included in typical benefits plans and the cost-savings implications of these options. Additionally, plan design options are presented including flexible benefits plans and self-funding options. The complexity of providing employee benefits has evolved over the decades to a point where both employers and employees have numerous options to consider. It is important, therefore, that each organization custom design its plan to meet its own needs. Flexibility is a key component.

The recent upheavals in the delivery and financing of health care have shifted focus away from indemnity plans to managed care. Managed care, the latest watchword in cost management, has become synonymous with enrollment in a health maintenance organization type program. Chapter 4 provides an in-depth discussion of the ABCs of managed care. As the proliferation of managed care organizations continues, the key question remains unanswered: Does managed care contain costs? The implications of this new system are discussed, particularly in reference to economic and legal issues.

The twin issues of cost and quality are becoming linked in the minds of the consumers of care. It is no longer enough for managed care organizations to maximize cost savings. The purchasers of care are rightfully demanding documentation of both economic and noneconomic factors associated with the delivery of care. Little is known about how the changes taking place will affect health care costs, access and quality. As such, there is a need to define and measure outcomes of care. The rapid adoption of managed care, one of the most significant changes to health care financing and delivery, has unknown consequences for patients, providers and health care organizations. Chapter 5 focuses on the importance of ensuring quality of care in the age of managed care. Discussion focuses on issues surrounding quality management and the means of assessing quality, patient satisfaction and outcomes research. Managed care organizations realize that data on these factors are key. Focus now is on managing, not just treating. The market is rapidly becoming data driven, and managed care companies prosper or die on their documented ability to contain costs without sacrificing quality of care.

Just about all would agree that most of us would be healthier if we took better care of ourselves. Years of poor health habits are a tremendous drain on the health care system and contribute to employee absenteeism, failure to work at full potential and lost productivity. Ironically, almost all of the risk factors identified with the major causes of sickness and death are behavioral or have a large behavioral component on which technology-intensive medicine has limited impact. The values of the "new" health care system must become oriented more toward prevention rather than cure, toward behavioral rather than purely medical/surgical care, and toward individual participation in the process of staying well. Chapter 6 focuses on wellness and health promotion and how these programs can be integrated into an organization's benefits plan. Discussion explores the importance of health promotion as well as the costs and benefits of wellness programs, which do have the potential to be a major factor in containing health care costs.

The costs of mental illnesses and substance abuse are staggering, and the situation is too widespread to ignore. Most companies and trust funds face the prospect of many employees being addicted to alcohol or drugs at some point during their employment. Lost worker productivity, increased accidents, absenteeism, employee theft and medical claims are just some of the adverse effects of substance abuse at the workplace. Chapter 7 focuses on the high costs of substance abuse. Highlighted in this chapter is the extent of substance abuse problems among the workforce, the costs associated with such abuse and options to be considered. It is shown that direct and indirect costs are substantial and the employer's ability to manage these costs is not easily accomplished.

The high financial and personal costs of workers' compensation are discussed in Chapter 8. Work-related injuries and illnesses are increasing, and the costs associated with these incidents are not insignificant. Just as employers have tried to be cost efficient in managing health care costs, it is imperative that attention be paid to workers' compensation and disability costs. The importance of prompt rehabilitation of the injured worker and the need to ferret out fraud and abuse is stressed. Workplace safety programs are very effective and important to implement. Discussion also focuses on the emergence of managed workers' compensation, which applies the techniques of managed care to work-related injuries and diseases.

The aging of America is making eldercare a huge workplace issue. Chapter 9 focuses on the costs of retiree benefits and how employers are addressing this politically and legally charged issue. Retiree health benefits have emerged as one of the most difficult problems in the employee benefits field. As the baby boom generation approaches retirement age, the potential costs for this benefit could be staggering. The legal ramifications of reducing and/or terminating health insurance coverage for retirees is reviewed, as are the implications of the Financial Accounting Standard (FAS) Ruling 106, which recognizes obligations for past service liabilities on the balance sheet and initially sent shock waves through the business community. Also included is discussion on long-term care and home care, two huge issues which must be addressed in light of the projected insolvency of the Medicare trust fund.

As the field of employee benefits/human resources gets more complicated, it is imperative that employers and employees have the information they need to make intelligent decisions. Since employee benefits constitute an ever-growing proportion of employees' total compensation and consume a large part of an employer's payroll, it behooves every employer to establish excellent communication programs to educate their employees about the value of their benefits package and the need to eliminate unnecessary, costly care and to become more cost-conscious consumers.

Providing a benefit does not automatically guarantee that employees will use it or use it properly. If a cost-effective health plan is to be successful, one must have an informed employee population. It won't work otherwise. Therefore, it is extremely important to make sure that the benefits literature delineates in an easy-to-understand manner benefits offerings and options. An evaluation/assessment strategy to monitor what is working and what is not is imperative as well. Chapter 10 focuses on the means of evaluation and communication. How does one select a managed care plan? How does one know if the changes made are meeting the objectives of the organization? The flood of data often can be confusing and conflicting, not to mention overwhelming. Evaluation, however, is a prerequisite for any plan redesign.

Chapter 11 tries to tie together the themes of the book. The field has become much more complex and there are more options to consider. The central message, however, is timeless: Know what your cost problems are. Health care costs are influenced both by price increases (which have been abating somewhat recently) and the number of medical tests and procedures performed (which have been increasing somewhat recently). The factors influencing health costs are numerous, but a cost-conscious consumer will be able to navigate his or her way if decisions are made intelligently (i.e., don't make decisions in a vacuum). Evaluate and assess, then implement measures that will save money but not adversely affect quality of care. Leave your options open; be prepared to modify or eliminate strategies that are not working. Most importantly, don't be complacent—you can't afford to be!

CHAPTER 1

What Ails Our System

For decades, the American health care system was controlled by the providers of care. It was the physician who would decide when a patient would be admitted to the hospital, which tests and procedures would be performed, and how long the patient would remain in the hospital. The physician's judgment was unquestioned. Given that an individual's health insurance policy covered most of the costs of care, the patient rarely had to worry about how he or she was going to afford the care rendered. But, over the decades, the synergism of a complex mix of social, political and economic forces has created an unwieldy, inefficient system. The enormous cost of health care now threatens efforts to balance the federal budget and is adversely affecting the bottom line of most businesses. While the current problems with the system are evident even to the most casual observer, the solutions are far from obvious. Looking back in time, however, one can see many missed opportunities for reform.

As the economics of health care has assumed a more prominent role in the delivery of health care, both management and labor have come to realize that failure to achieve a more disciplined health care system has serious financial implications not only for their industry, but for the nation as a whole. The costs of providing health benefits are no longer an incidental cost of doing business. Organizations are forced to allocate an ever-increasing share of their operating expenses to fund benefit packages and consequently must raise prices, reduce profits or both.

The changes which have taken place over the past decades have been nothing short of astounding. Yet, many of the current problems can be traced to earlier times. Indeed, the seeds of the system's current problems took root decades ago. Paul Starr's *The Social Transformation of American Medicine* is a particularly excellent source to gain a better appreciation of what was. What will be is anyone's guess!

This chapter will review the policies that helped shape the health care system and show how past actions laid the foundation for the cost crisis of the latter half of this century. Discussion will focus on the shift in the loci of power, control and influence away from the physician/organized medicine to a market-driven, for-profit bureaucracy more concerned with the bottom line. It is maintained herein that, of the numerous transitions in the delivery and financing of health care in the United States during the 20th century, the supremacy of the managed health care conglomerates over organized medicine is one of the most significant.

Depression Years

Attention to rising medical costs first became an issue in the years preceding and immediately following the Depression. Medical care was a bigger item in family medical budgets than wage losses, illustrating that higher costs of medical care (physician services and hospital care) were an important concern. For many, hospital charges plus physician bills for in-hospital services could represent as much as 40% of total family medical expenditures. The costs of physician care rose because of improved quality and increasing monopoly power. In general, hospital charges were still relatively low so less attention was paid to these costs or the problems of hospital reimbursement.

Despite this situation, efforts to establish a form of health insurance failed. Physicians were generally unenthusiastic about the prospect, and the American Federation of Labor opposed any program characterizing compulsory health insurance as an unnecessary, paternalistic reform that would create a system of state supervision of the people's health. Samuel Gompers worried that a government insurance system would weaken unions by usurping their role in providing social benefits. Employers, too, viewed compulsory health insurance as contrary to their interests. They did not want any competition from government in social welfare programs. Hence, the three main protagonists—the medical profession, unions and business—had rejected the concept, each for their own self-serving reasons.

Although reform initiatives were rejected, there was a realization that the health cost crisis had to be addressed in some manner. The Committee on the Costs of Medical Care, a privately funded commission, was formed to study medical policy issues. The committee issued comprehensive reports on medical care in America from 1928-1932. Recommendations included reducing economic barriers to medical care and organizing it on a bureaucratic model and turning over power to the professionals. Compulsory health insurance was opposed.

The New Deal Years

The New Deal era saw a shift toward social reform. The Roosevelt administration achieved great success in this area, but decided to sidestep the issue of health care insurance even though during this time period it was difficult for many to pay for medical services. Physicians' incomes suffered as a result, and hospitals were in similar trouble. Beds were empty, bills were unpaid and utilization fell. Federal emergency relief funds were made available, but that was as far as the administration was willing to go.

Although a national health insurance bill was not enacted, the private sector stepped in to fill the void. During the 1930s, Blue Cross and Blue Shield plans were formed. Blue Cross actually started against the advice of those in the insurance industry because the actuaries did not believe that they could predict losses with confidence. They were wrong. The experience of Blue Cross' success defied expectations, and soon the commercial carriers followed suit and began offering indemnity coverage against hospital expenses on a group basis. Although Blue Cross had tax exemption status and privileged relations with hospitals, the commercial carriers' larger financial resources and relationships with the employers propelled their growth.

Postwar Years

Private health insurance, which began to grow during the 1930s, proliferated during the 1940s. Concomitant with this growth was the variation in third party involvement with providers and differences in coverage. The American Medical Association (AMA), however, insisted that all health insurance plans accept the private physicians' monopoly control of the medical market and complete authority over all aspects of medical institutions. Under this system, providers were reimbursed on a fee-for-service basis.

Postwar expansion was a boon to the commercial insurers and, as the commercial insurers grew, the character of the industry changed. The commercial market was selling more policies than the Blue Cross Blue Shield plans. The most attractive aspect of the commercial carriers was that they were willing to give employers a lower price on healthy, low-risk workers. Whereas Blue Cross subscribers paid the same community rate, under commercial insurance every employee group was charged according to its experience. As the costs of medical care increased, the Blues raised the share of the costs borne directly by the consumer. Not surprisingly, the number of subscribers fell. So, even though the Blues pioneered the feasibility of providing health insurance, the way the market evolved, they were left holding the bag, so to speak. The commercial insurers picked off the low-risk employees and left the high-cost population to the Blues. Competition forced the Blues to adopt experience rating, but the commercial carriers continued to have the advantage.

Meanwhile, during the 1940s, the issue of universal and comprehensive health insurance reform was ping-ponged in the halls of Congress. Instead of a single health insurance system for the entire population, a system of private insurance for those who could afford it and public welfare services for the poor emerged. President Truman called upon Congress to pass a national program to assure the right to adequate medical care and protection from the economic ramifications of sickness. Predictably, the AMA was opposed to the plan as were most other health care interests. Reform failed yet again, which meant that health insurance in America would be predominantly private.

Post-World War II saw the emergence of unions' bargaining leverage on behalf of their members. The consumer had little organized influence in medical care affairs but, once the unions began bargaining collectively with management over health care, the former became a significant influence on the services received by their members as well as on the medical system as a whole. Actually, the unions' struggle for influence in welfare programs was one of their few political successes during this period. Labor managed to secure and expand fringe benefit packages in the absence of wage increases; i.e., pension plans, insurance and vacation time became part of the collective bargaining agreement. It was welfare bargaining as much as any other subject that brought about the Taft-Hartley Act of 1948.

The Taft-Hartley Act created jointly managed employee benefit trust funds. These welfare and pension funds are the principal means by which private industry covered all unionized workers and their dependents. These funds became key intermediaries in financing health care for workers in the construction, coal mining and service industries. Under this arrangement, several employers are able to make a financial contribution to a central fund, thereby spreading the risk over the entire group. The larger employers were given more of an interest in controlling the costs of health care, since they were committed to pay for a level of benefits, regardless of the cost. This situation would become a powerful element in the politics of American health care.

In summary, a review of the history of the first half of the 20th century shows that political forces served to torpedo efforts to create a national health insurance system despite economic factors which clearly showed that such a system would have benefited much of the population. The middle class bought private insurance, the unions began to look to collective bargaining for health benefits and the poor were taken care of in charity hospitals. The modern medical care system was evolving into one in which independent physicians were reimbursed on a fee-for-service payment system, independent hospitals were paid essentially on a cost-reimbursement basis and patients were insured by third party intermediaries. Each component was interdependent; each responded within the limits and incentives offered by the economic framework of the system.

For years the system operated in a symbiotic manner with the hospitals competing for doctors who brought in the patients, and each was reimbursed by third parties without question. Under this arrangement, however, the third parties had no serious leverage over the costs generated by the hospitals or the physicians. The premiums and charges reflected the cost-generating behavior of the providers in his or her community and the experience of the insured group. Payments were made on the basis of usual, customary and reasonable charges.

Under this system of private insurance, the providers benefited greatly. The blank check nature of the system did little to encourage the cost-effective delivery of care. Since reimbursement for care was part of the fringe benefits, and not an out-of-pocket expense, there was no incentive for individuals to reduce spending or even care about the costs of care. In sum, insurance, as it had been applied to health care, caused a massive distortion in the delivery and economics of health services. The system did little to help those who were retired, out of work, self-employed, or employed but not offered health benefits. Millions of poor and chronically ill could not get health insurance. Those who purchased health insurance on their own had to pay more for the same coverage than those who received it as a fringe benefit. This inequity set the stage for the debate to come.

The Formative Years: The 1960s

During the second half of the century, the health care system changed dramatically. The explosion in technology and research created a powerful medical industry. Organized medicine was a powerful force and dictated the way medical care would be delivered. Expansion of hospital building increased the number of beds tremendously. Also, there was an expansion in the number of medical schools and in the number of students studying medicine. An immense new system of medical schools, teaching hospitals and other health-related institutions was created. New power bases were formed. All of these factors contributed to the restructuring of the system.

During the 1960s, the push for reform was embodied in the Great Society legislative agenda. The social programs of the 1960s were aimed at alleviating poverty, and the health programs addressed the issues of insuring the poor and aged. The movement for a contributory insurance program for the elderly and the poor, culminating in the passage of Medicare and Medicaid in 1965, to this day has far-reaching implications for the delivery and financing of health care. Medicare, enacted as part of the Social Security Act of 1965, was the first nationwide, federally funded health insurance program for the elderly. The intent was to provide financial assistance to individuals during their non-income-earning years. Medicare Part A pays for skilled nursing, home health agencies, and hospice and dialysis services. Part B, Medicare's voluntary part, covers doctor bills and other outpatient expenses and is financed by general tax revenue and monthly premiums paid by beneficiaries. Medicaid is the joint federal/state-administered program through which low-income individuals who meet income/assets requirements obtain health services. Some have said that we are haunted by the political accommodations made in the early 1960s to get these bills enacted.

Primarily to gain the cooperation of the doctors and hospitals, the bill stipulated that fiscal intermediaries, the private insurance carriers and the Blues, would provide reimbursement, although the federal government was to pay the bills. Under this system, the federal government surrendered direct control of the program and its costs. Another key component of the legislation was that hospitals would be paid according to their costs rather than a schedule of negotiated rates. This arrangement turned out to be extremely favorable to the providers.

Cracks in the Foundation: The 1970s

Over the next decades, the rise in health care expenditures steadily increased. Public dissatisfaction increased with the rising costs. A survey taken in 1970 found that three-quarters of those polled believed that there was a crisis in health care in the United States. The ever-evolving health care system was not working efficiently. It was fragmented, costly, inefficient and poorly managed. The poor were still not receiving adequate medical care. There was a maldistribution of physicians across the country. There were too many hospital beds. Not helping matters was the very real presence of persistent inflation and an economic recession. The Nixon administration imposed a freeze on wages and prices. This Economic Stabilization Program (ESP) went into effect in 1971 through 1974. Post-ESP, from 1975-1977, a series of Medicare amendments was passed in an effort to control both utilization of hospital services as well as Medicare hospital outlays.

Section 222 supported incentive reimbursement demonstrations, voluntary and mandatory rate setting programs, alternative care demonstrations and approaches to cost containment. Section 223 gave Medicare the authority to disallow any costs unnecessary to the efficient provision of care. Also, *professional standards review organizations (PSROs)* were established to monitor quality of federally funded care and to ensure its delivery in a cost-efficient manner. Section 223 was later amended in 1979 to implement total cost limits. These changes laid the groundwork for the prospective payment system enacted in 1983. Meanwhile, new forces gradually emerged to change the system. The concept of a national health insurance program once again was raised.

During the 1970s and 1980s, medical costs rose sharply and the government's share of the costs increased significantly. Many attributed the rising costs to Medicare and Medicaid. In reality, Medicare and Medicaid only reinforced the basic incentives in the existing health care system. The key problem was the financing arrangements. The fee-for-service insurance system had few incentives for either the provider or the patient to minimize the cost of treatment. The insurer's role was simply to forecast expenditures, determine risk, collect premiums and pay the bills. Both private insurers and the government's programs insulated patients and providers alike from the costs of services. First dollar coverage was common. The structure of financing and reimbursement was designed to encourage higher costs. Providers, perversely, were encouraged to maximize reimbursements. There was an absence of any effective restraints. Medicaid was draining state and local governments' budgets; Medicare was draining the federal budget. While the government began squeezing the providers by capping reimbursement rates, the providers responded by shifting costs to those covered by insurance. Employers and insurers began to retaliate by initiating cost-containment strategies.

The politics of health care post-1970 is a study unto itself. Special interest groups were sufficiently strong to block almost any coherent course of action. Numerous regulations served to strangle the system. The skewed incentives of the reimbursement system were left unchanged while new layers of controls were added. In response, or perhaps out of frustration, employers and the insurance carriers initiated their own cost-containment strategies to address the cost crisis. But in order to fully understand and appreciate how employers and providers provided the impetus for changes in the health care system, it is necessary to digress and briefly review the expansion of employee benefits.

Expansion of Employee Benefits

Employee benefits systems represented an important part of an employer's total compensation package and could be categorized into two broad groups: compensation for time not worked (such as paid holidays, vacations and sick leave) and nonwage compensation. The latter refers to benefits that are legislatively mandated (such as Social Security premiums, unemployment compensation and workers' compensation) or benefits that are contractual agreements between employers and employees, including pensions (which are the largest component of nonwage benefits) and insurance. The substantial growth over time in nonwage compensation is the result of federal legislation creating Medicare, expanding coverage of the Social Security system to include almost all workers, raising the salary base on which employers are to pay Social Security taxes and increasing the Social Security tax rate. Certain benefits help the employee meet special needs and are tax exempt (health care, for example); others are tax deferred (retirement income employee benefit programs, for example). Many benefits are required by law (employer contributions to Social Security, Medicare, workers' compensation insurance and unemployment insurance, for example); others are voluntary.

The employee benefits system in America is a voluntary system in the sense that it is without federal requirements dictating how an organization must establish an employee benefit plan (pension, health and/or welfare benefits). This is not to imply that the system is unregulated. Indeed, employee benefit plans have been subjected to a stream of legislative activity, which has created a complex web of constraints and requirements with which the plans must comply in order to maintain a tax-favored status. The tax treatment of employee benefit programs has been consistent over time: Health insurance contributions by employers are tax exempt, and retirement and capital accumulation programs are tax deferred. Whereas relatively favorable tax treatment of employee benefits has been an impetus for employers to provide such benefits rather than paying employees higher wages, the growth of these benefits occurred at the expense of wage and salary income, which contributes to the tax base.

From the 1940s through the mid-1970s, congressional actions focused on providing protection of benefits to participants. This permitted the growth of employee benefit programs, reflecting a commitment to provide security to active workers, disabled workers, and retirees and their families. Probably one of the most far-reaching pieces of legislation was the Employee Retirement Income Security Act (ERISA) of 1974. Prior to ERISA, the U.S. benefits system was substantially unregulated. ERISA was designed to protect the pension and welfare rights of workers covered by private pension plans. Among its major provisions were the establishment of minimum participation standards with regard to age and length of service, the funding of annual costs of pension plans and the systematic amortization of accumulated unfunded pension liabilities. The appendix summarizes the basic tenets of the act.

ERISA also led to an unbundling of the risk and administrative functions of insurers, which spurred the growth of self-insurance. By exempting self-insured plans from state regulation of health insurance, ERISA gave strong financial rewards to self-insured employers. Self-insured plans were not subject to state laws requiring health plans to provide specified benefits mandated by state legislation; self-insured plans were also not subject to state premium taxes. Self-insurance allowed firms to pay claims as they were submitted, rather than paying an insurance premium; hence employers were able to earn interest on their working capital.

There was little self-insurance in the mid-1970s but, thanks to ERISA, nearly one decade later more than two-thirds of the nation's employees with conventional coverage were enrolled in a plan with some aspects of self-insurance. Self-insured companies logically did not need the services of the Blues or commercial insurance companies to insure financial risk. New vendors, *third party administrators (TPAs),* were formed to fill the void. TPAs specialized in providing administrative services without additional expenses incurred with underwriting costs. In order to still capture some of this new market, the commercial carriers and the Blues offered *administrative services only* or partial insurance protection called *minimum premium* or *stop-loss plans.* The growth of TPAs was tremendous during the 1970s.

In addition to ERISA, subsequent pieces of legislation addressed the ways employee benefits were funded and administered. From TEFRA (Tax Equity and Fiscal Responsibility Act of 1982) to DEFRA (Deficit Reduction Act of 1984) to COBRA (Consolidated Omnibus Budget Reconciliation Act of 1985) to the much hated and soon-repealed Section 89 of the Internal Revenue Code as part of the Tax Reform Act of 1986, congressional actions gave form and substance to the way employee benefits were designed and administered. In one sense, Congress created an environment in which benefit plans are costly and very difficult to administer.

Since the mid-1980s, benefit costs have escalated not only because of the costs of new programs, but also because of the spiraling costs of maintaining compliance with existing benefit plans. Whereas social policy appeared to influence the nature and scope of benefits packages prior to the 1980s, since that time revenue considerations appear to have dictated the types of benefits offered. Plans became more comprehensive, complex and costly. The halcyon days of past decades were over, and cost containment and better management of the benefits package was essential.

The Era of Health Care Cost Containment: The 1980s and Beyond

Previously, it was rare for employers to consider seriously the cost of providing health and medical benefits to employees. The cost of health care was not overwhelming; there was no need to be concerned with cost management. Escalating costs of employer-provided benefits and insurance premiums furnished the impetus for the private and public sectors to do something about the costs of employee health benefits.

On October 1, 1983, Medicare replaced its cost-based system of reimbursement for hospitals with prospective payment. Hospitals would receive a rate fixed in advance for each admission rather than receive payment for the costs actually incurred. The rate depended on the patient's diagnostic related group (DRG) code and on certain characteristics of the hospital. Additionally, the peer review organizations were empowered to review admissions. Analysis found, however, that while there was a decline in admissions, it was a result of the review system and not of the prospective rates.

The Medicare program is in serious financial difficulty 15 years after prospective payment primarily because a larger group of citizens are eligible for an expanded program, because costs are rising much faster than overall inflation, because we are living longer and consuming more health care goods and services, and because of an increase in those younger than age 65 with disabilities who qualify for Social Security and also qualify for Medicare Part A benefits. The trust fund for the federal hospital insurance program (Medicare Part A), which derives most of its income from payroll taxes, is projected to be exhausted in 2002. Costs are rising rapidly in Part B, too, but because the financing mechanism for Part B is different, bankruptcy is not an issue.

Also during the 1980s there was a shift in reimbursement for physician services. Medicare's customary, prevailing and reasonable payment system was, by consensus, unsatisfactory. The system was inflationary and slow to respond to technological changes. A Medicare fee freeze was implemented; however, three years after the freeze went into effect, beneficiaries were spending almost 30% more for physician services, primarily for surgery, diagnostic testing and radiology. Other methods were needed to contain costs.

A new fee schedule system, *resource-based relative value scale (RBRVS)*, was formulated and implemented in 1992. Under RBRVS, a relative value for each procedure was assigned, and there were a geographic adjustment factor and a dollar conversion factor. The RBRVS takes into account physician behavior including price and volume of services in an effort to establish greater control over expenditures. It was believed that RBRVS could serve as a rational foundation for compensating physicians according to the work and effort they exert in performing services. However, the ascendancy of managed care has superseded the way physicians are reimbursed and will be discussed in Chapter 4.

The goal of cost containment during the 1980s was to lower both unnecessary expenditures and inappropriate utilization. It was believed that the key to managing costs was to provide alternatives to costly medical services such as hospital care. The focus was on reducing the total number of admissions and average lengths of stay. Outpatient care was strongly encouraged. Early cost-containment strategies focused on utilization review, which included preadmission testing, utilization review, second surgical opinion programs, higher coinsurance and lower deductibles, wellness programs, and hospital bill audits. Utilization review (UR) generally refers to the monitoring of appropriateness, necessity, quantity and quality of health care. In the past, the focus of UR was quality assurance. That is, the medical sector developed self-policing mechanisms such as hospital issue committees. More recently, however, the focus has shifted to cost control, with the medical community superseded by the payers of health care in implementing UR.

Hindsight shows that there are no simple solutions to the cost problem. While a variety of incentives to hold down costs were tried, health care costs continued to rise. Part of the problem stemmed from the fact that there was no unanimity of opinion as to what constituted a cost-effective package. What may have worked for one organization would not necessarily work for another. Employers tried a variety of incentives to hold down costs, which can be grouped into two broad classes: consumer incentives and provider incentives (depending upon whether the incentives act directly on the consumer or provider behavior).

In frustration (or desperation) most employers focused on implementing higher deductibles and employee contributions. The percent of employees whose health insurance premiums were wholly paid by the employers declined significantly. However, increasing the portion of expenses borne by employees may have saved money for the employer, but did not reduce overall expenditures. The employer was treating the symptoms, not the disease. Total health care costs continued to increase, as did the volume and intensity of services. While in-hospital utilization declined, the cost of a hospital stay soared. While the rate of inpatient surgery decreased, the cost of outpatient surgery soared. Although the rate of office visits slowed, the ordering of diagnostic tests increased. Managing health care costs had never been more frustrating.

The Conception of Managed Care:
The Beginning or the End?

In response to the events of the day, a new form of delivery system emerged: the prepaid group practice or *health maintenance organization (HMO)*. The conservative Republican administration encouraged private initiatives and believed that the HMO represented a more efficient form of management. The HMO Act of 1972 established regulations and qualification standards for HMOs. Under this system, a physician serves as the primary care physician, who coordinates health care. These "gatekeepers" are counted on to prevent excessive use of the health care system without theoretically denying necessary treatment. The early HMOs employed physicians (staff model). Over time, HMOs have evolved into *individual practice associations (IPAs)* in which an administrative and management group contracts with independent physicians to deliver care. The HMO collects premiums and pays the provider according to a schedule based primarily on actual utilization. IPA doctors see patients in their own offices. Under a group model HMO, physicians are partners in a group practice and their compensation is directly dependent on the financial success of the HMO. There is a strong incentive to provide cost-effective treatment and to curtail unnecessary services.

HMOs have been successful in controlling hospital costs and utilization. But the larger question is, do they contain overall health care costs? This question will be discussed in the chapter on managed care. Along with the rise in the HMO was the creation of the *PPO (preferred provider organization)*. Under the PPO concept, providers offer negotiated discounts from normal fees to participants who elect to use their services. They range from local arrangements between a single hospital and a single employer to a large, sophisticated organization that includes many hospitals, doctors and employers. As with HMOs, an essential element of a successful PPO is the ability to identify efficient health care providers who provide quality care at reasonable cost. Ironically, as PPOs evolved during the 1980s, they became more like HMOs. However, unlike HMOs, PPOs are not regulated. There are no standards in place. There is also little information showing that the PPO networks and hybrid PPOs provide savings. There are still many problems to be worked out to ensure that quality will not suffer. There is no assurance of the adequacy of these networks and the credentials of the providers. Again, the chapter on managed care will address these issues in greater detail.

The creation and growth of the HMO and PPO signaled the beginning of the corporatization of the health care system. Indeed, the 1980s and 1990s saw the beginnings of another transformation of the health care system. Competition was encouraged in an effort to stem costs and reform the system. Unlike the past, this time the physicians' loss of autonomy, control and power seemed more permanent. Power was amassing in the hands of huge health care chains, conglomerates and holding companies. These entities, not the physicians or organized medicine, were propelling changes in the way health care was to be delivered and financed. Cost efficiency fueled the move to integrate and centralize. Physicians were being forced to choose a more cost-efficient manner of practice in order to survive. Employer corporations were intent on selecting only the most cost-efficient health insurers and providers.

Starr outlined five dimensions distinguishing the growth of corporate medicine:

1. Change in the type of ownership and control; a shift from the non-profit and governmental organizations to for-profit companies
2. The decline of freestanding institutions and the rise of multi-institutional systems
3. Diversification and corporate restructuring; shift to conglomerates
4. Shift from acute care hospitals to organizations such as HMOs that embrace the various phases and levels of care
5. Mergers and acquisitions; industry concentration of ownership and control in regional markets and the nation as a whole.

The rise of corporate health care is one of the most significant consequences of the changing structure of medical care. Indeed, establishing standards of proper medical care, focusing on lower cost alternatives and more efficient practice styles, and setting criteria for appropriateness are all noble goals. But, with this solidification in the market has come micromanagement. New layers of bureaucrats have been added to police the providers. The system's efficiency is compromised by the fragmented, complex payment system.

The Call for Reform . . . Yet Again

Once again, health care reform has emerged as a critical issue in America. Escalating costs, increasing insurance burdens on employers, an inefficient administrative structure and the growing number of uninsured have created a national mandate for change. The Clinton administration's proposal to radically change the way health care is delivered and financed came at a time when people were calling for reform. Rising out-of-pocket costs and fear of losing one's health insurance coverage were the two interrelated factors that provided the impetus for reform. The principles advocated in the Clinton proposal could not be faulted: Security (mandating universal coverage), quality, choice, responsibility, simplicity (bringing uniformity to the day-to-day administration of the system) and savings were sensible and important objectives, but the obstacles to successful passage of the Health Security Act of 1993 could not be overcome. Unfortunately, efforts to reform the system failed primarily because of naivety and intense lobbying on behalf of the key players.

Scores of other health reform proposals were introduced into Congress, ranging from minor changes to the present system to those calling for a universal health insurance system. Just as call for reform met with defeat in the Roosevelt, Truman and Nixon administrations, the Clinton administration could not surmount the political pressures. President Johnson managed to effect change with the passage of Medicare and Medicaid, but most will argue that the political compromises he had to make to achieve passage are haunting us now. Meanwhile, the managed care industry has succeeded in transforming the system to comply with its objectives.

Summary

The social, political and economic forces over the past decades have served to mold and shape the U.S. health care system, and events of the past certainly contributed to—if not laid the foundation for—the health care crisis of the latter part of the century. Over time we have witnessed the rise and decline of organized medicine's power and control over the way health care is delivered and financed. We have seen the rise of the third party insurance system with its blank check reimbursement strategy insulate the consumers from the cost of the product they were purchasing. We have seen the rise in employee benefits with employers paying insurance premiums and employees having no idea how much they cost. Since insurance premiums are tax free, workers often received more generous insurance with lower deductibles and broader coverage. We have seen the evolution and tremendous growth in the self-insurance market, which has eroded the third party system's power. We have seen an unprecedented rise of a huge health care bureaucracy which, as of this writing, seems to be calling the shots. Hence, what was once a cottage industry has been transformed into a "medical industrial complex" with special interest groups trying to capture as much of the market as possible.

There have been many opportunities to enact universal health insurance reform, but each time coalitions served to block its passage. What has materialized over time is a system that is terribly fragmented, complex and costly.

One does not have to be an economist to realize that the fundamental principles of the marketplace do not apply to health care. The laws of supply and demand never worked in the health marketplace; providers create their own demand. In contrast to the way people buy most other products and services, they do little comparison shopping for medical treatments. The patient/consumer depends on the doctor to decide what treatment is needed, which hospital to be admitted to, which drugs to prescribe. Unlike just about every other thing a consumer spends money on, there is no limit on what they will pay for health. That someone else is paying the bill significantly contributes to the Alice in Wonderland environment.

As debate continues on how the health care system should be reconfigured, there are sharply differing diagnoses of the problem and the prescriptions for its reform. We know how we got ourselves into this morass; we do not agree on how to get out of it.

APPENDIX

Employee Retirement Income Security Act of 1974

The Employee Retirement Income Security Act of 1974 (ERISA) is the major piece of legislation affecting the private pension system. It also set in motion subsequent pieces of legislation designed to accommodate new developments or correct flaws in earlier legislation.

The chief purpose of ERISA was to protect the interests of workers and their beneficiaries. The act was instituted to ensure:

- That workers and employees are not required to satisfy unreasonable age and service requirements before they can be eligible to participate in an employer- or fund-sponsored pension plan
- That individuals who work for a specified minimum period while covered by a pension plan receive at least some pension at retirement through vesting, benefit accrual and break-in-service provisions
- That pension promises are adequately funded by establishing minimum funding standards
- That the monies set aside to meet future pension promises are invested as a prudent person would invest. Plan trustees are made personally liable for breaches of fiduciary responsibility in the operation of the plan
- That employees and their beneficiaries know their rights under the plan by requiring employers to report and disclose plan provisions
- That the benefits promised through defined benefit plans are protected in the event of plan termination by establishing plan termination insurance
- That spouses of pensioners are protected through joint and survivor provisions.

Subsequent legislation was intended to refine ERISA or to address emerging situations. Another thrust of the subsequent legislation was to redefine and calibrate the relationship between defined benefit and defined contribution pension plans.

CHAPTER 2

Health Care Costs and the Effect on Employee Benefits

R arely does a day go by without a reference made in some newspaper, magazine or trade journal about the high cost of health care. Seminars on various aspects of health care cost management abound, and consulting companies specialize in trimming the fat from benefits packages. With the costs of health care continuously outstripping the growth in prices in the U.S. economy, the business community is increasingly concerned that their firms are being hurt in domestic and international markets. Employees are also concerned about the high costs of medical care since they are absorbing more of these costs. Union leaders are in a difficult position of protecting gains made in collective bargaining (during the 1980s, most labor disputes centered on health benefits).

Medical care in the United States is generally acknowledged to be among the best in the world. Physicians and other health personnel are highly trained and they command high fees for their services. It is also common knowledge that the United States spends more on health care than any other nation but does not rank as high on key morbidity and mortality indicators. Both infant mortality and life expectancy are traditional key indicators of health status. Access to care, too, is an indicator of the availability of services to the general population. Even though the United States spends most per capita for health care, it is not ranked in the top ten countries in infant mortality. Nor is it ranked in the top ten for life expectancy. Japan has the longest life expectancy and one of the lowest infant mortality rates; yet its per capita expenditure for health care is less than half that of the United States. There are over 40 million Americans who are uninsured; in every other developed nation, there is some form of national health insurance or a national health service.

Are Americans getting their money's worth? One could conclude that despite vast expenditures for health care, the U.S. system is providing neither universal access nor a higher health status that other nations enjoy for comparatively less money.

The amount spent on health services, supplies, research and construction absorbs nearly one-seventh of the aggregate output of the U.S. economy. Primarily due to the continued and rapid growth in personal health care expenditures, anxiety and concern about future health care spending has increased. Both individuals and state and federal governments are struggling with rising costs. This chapter focuses on the cost of health care including the growth in expenditures, contributing factors to this growth, and the implications for businesses and trust funds. It will be shown that other developed countries' costs have not risen as rapidly and that the health of their population is not being jeopardized.

Trends in U.S. Health Care Expenditures

The trend in rising U.S. health care costs is multifaceted, and the synergy among the forces driving the increase further complicates matters. Spending for national health care has increased steadily in dollar terms as well as in proportion of the Gross Domestic Product (GDP). The GDP measures the output of U.S. economy as the market value of goods and services produced within its geographic boundaries. The share of the nation's resources spent on health care has increased an average of .3% of the GDP per year since 1960. To illustrate the point better, whereas the average annual expenditures per consumer unit increased by 3% from 1992 to 1993, there was a 9% increase in expenditures for health care during this same time period. Health care expenditures take a big bite out of our pockets and have done so for decades.

National health care expenditures (hospital, physician and dental services; nursing home care; drugs; and medical supplies) increased from $23.9 billion in 1960 to over $884.2 billion in 1993, representing 13.9% of the GDP. The 1993 figure is 7.8% higher than that for 1992. Although health expenditures grew at the slowest rates since 1986, spending is still increasing faster than the overall economy. In fact, since 1980, health spending has been the second fastest growing component of the federal budget. Only the interest costs of the mounting public debt have risen more quickly. Without any reform, health care expenditures are projected to rise by an average annual rate of growth of 13.5% over the next five years. It is projected that the cost of health care will rise from 14% of the GDP in 1994 to 18% in the year 2000. In dollar amounts, it is projected that $1 trillion will be spent on health care in the year 2000. That is, without reform, in less than ten years, almost $1 of every $5 will go to cover the costs of health care!

While no single factor explains why health care spending has grown as fast as it has, there are several influences that collectively contribute to the situation. In particular, increases over the last several years have been primarily the result of

- Medical inflation, which accounted for a large portion of the growth during the 1980s and 1990s, and increased spending on health insurance. For example, the 10% increase in health insurance expenditures in 1993 followed increases of 11% and 13% in the two prior years, respectively. Expenditures on medical services and drugs rose 8% and 4%, respectively, during the same time period.
- The aging of the population, which added to health spending because older people tend to incur more health expenses per person than younger people
- Health care personnel's wages playing catch-up. Health care is labor-intensive and wages for nurses, doctors and other health personnel have risen faster than the average earnings of private, nonfarm workers.
- Medical technology. Sophisticated technology carries a big price tag, and the steady stream of new products and procedures adds to health care spending.

The rapid pace of increases in federal health spending complicates resolution of the federal budget deficits. Total federal spending in 1990, for example, would have been $50 billion *less* had health spending during the 1980s grown at the average rate of increase for all federal outlays.

Where the Health Care Dollars Went

During the past three decades, the system for funding health care services has evolved from one relying on direct patient out-of-pocket payment to that relying on third party private and government insurance programs. Whereas in 1960 direct out-of-pocket payments accounted for 55.9% of personal health care expenditures and third party private health insurance and government funding accounted for 22.6% and 21.4%, respectively, by the early 1990s, direct out-of-pocket funding declined to 21.4% while third party private payers' portion increased to 33.3%. The share of government funding grew to 45.3%, primarily due to the large increase in Medicare and Medicaid expenditures. Medicare and Medicaid spent $272.1 billion for health care in 1993, accounting for 30.8% of health spending and 70.2% of all public funding of health care. Fueling this spiral is an aggregate increase in the number of beneficiaries and an increase in costs per beneficiary.

Almost 89% of total national health expenditures was for personal health care services and products. In 1993, personal health expenditures grew to $782.5 billion, an increase of 7.2% from 1992. Personal health care expenditures were the greatest for hospital care and physician services. Expenditures for hospital care services topped $326.6 billion in 1993, representing 41.7% of the total $884.2 billion. The hospital share of personal health care expenditures increased substantially from 1960 to 1980, accounting for 38.9% ($3.9 billion) in 1960 and 46.7% ($102.4 billion) 20 years later. By 1993, the share of hospital expenditures dipped to 41.7% because of the shift to outpatient care facilities.

Physician expenditures, the second largest component of personal health care expenditures, declined from 22.2% ($5.3 billion) in 1960 to 19.1% ($41.9 billion) in 1980 only to rebound to 20.9% ($151.8 billion) in 1990 after the implementation of the prospective payment system. In 1993, $171.2 billion was spent on physician services, representing 21.9% of the total expenditures. Physician services have become a complement to and a substitute for hospital inpatient and outpatient care, and many services which had been performed on an inpatient basis have shifted to ambulatory settings.

Nursing home care expenditures increased from 4.2% ($1 billion) in 1960 to 9.1% ($20 billion) in 1980. Accounting for part of this growth is the fact that Medicaid nursing home benefits became available in 1973. The relative share of nursing home care remained fairly constant from 1980-1993, reaching $69.6 billion in 1993 and accounting for an estimated 8.9% of all personal health care expenditures. Figure 1 shows the percent distribution of personal health care expenditures by type of service from 1960 to 1993. Figures 2A and 2B show where the health care dollars came from and where they went.

Prices consumers pay for the most commonly prescribed prescription drugs continue to increase faster than the general inflation. The prices of these medications increased on average 4.3% from 1993-1994, while the general rate of inflation was 2.7% during this same time period. Manufacturers of these top selling prescription drugs earned profits far exceeding

FIGURE 1

Percent Distribution of Personal Health Care Expenditures by Type of Service

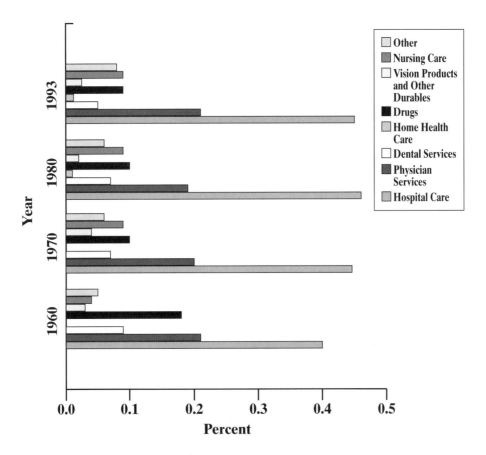

Source: Health Care Financing Administration data from the Office of the Actuary and the Office of National Cost Estimates.

those of other Fortune 500 companies. As an example, the price of Premarin, prescribed as an estrogen hormone replacement, increased 85% from 1989 to 1994. The price of Xanax, an antianxiety drug, increased 79%, and the price of Capoten, used to control high blood pressure, increased 65%. During this same time period, there were eight price increases for Premarin, and six for Xanax and Capoten, respectively. Not surprisingly, the manufacturers of these drugs have seen their profits soar. The median annual prof-

FIGURE 2A

The Nation's Health Dollar, 1993
Where It Came From

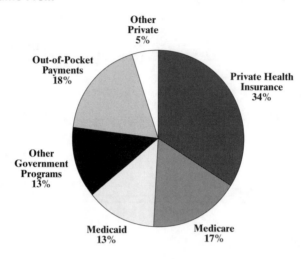

FIGURE 2B

The Nation's Health Dollar, 1993
Where It Went

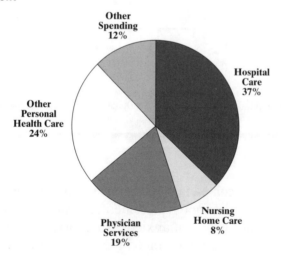

Source: Katherine R. Levit et al., Health Care Financing Review, Fall 1994.

it rate was 15% in 1993, which was more than five times higher than the median for all Fortune 500 companies in that year.

Spending for health care amounted to an estimated $3,299 per person in 1993, which is over three times greater than the average per capita expenditure in 1980 ($1,068) and ten times greater than the average outlay in 1970 ($346). Americans paid $157.5 billion out of pocket for personal health care services in 1993, a 4.6% increase from 1992. Out-of-pocket expenditures include copayments and deductibles, as well as direct payments for services and products not covered by third parties. These expenditures exclude private health insurance premiums.

Not surprisingly, there are variations in health care spending. The amount spent per capita on hospital care, physician services and prescription drugs varied tremendously by state and even between parts of the same state. Overall, New York and California accounted for one-fifth of all spending. Data show that what appears to be the most important factor influencing the level of health care spending in a state or an area is personal income. That is, those with high incomes tend to spend more on health care than those with low incomes. For example, New Englanders spent more for care than those living in the Rocky Mountain states but, when personal income was taken into account, spending as a share of personal income was approximately the same in both regions.

Other factors that influence cost variations include hospital bed capacity and number of physicians per capita. We know that provider practice patterns influence patient utilization rates as well as the services provided. Also, the cost of providing care will lead to variations. Those areas with high labor costs, high rent, medical malpractice premiums and bad debt percentages, for example, have higher cost ratios.

Age is an important factor. The Medicare program cost totaled $162 billion in 1994. Net Medicare spending per beneficiary is projected to grow at an average annual rate of 8.7% between 1995 and 2002, the year Medicare is projected to run out of money. Proportionately, the elderly devote the largest share of their total expenditures to health care (16%). Spending on health care by the youngest age group (younger than 25 years) decreased by 16% in 1993, and this group spent the least ($349) and devoted the smallest share of their total expenditures to health care (2%). The largest increase in health care spending (17%) was among those age 75 and older. This group spent the most on average ($2,883) on health care in 1993. Overall, 70% of Medicare funding is spent on only 10% of beneficiaries, with 20% of these beneficiaries spending in the last year of life.

Logically, states with the highest proportions of their population older than age 65 tend to have the highest health care costs. Florida, for example, traditionally has had the highest health care costs. Among the regions of the country, New England and the Middle Atlantic states had the highest per capita spending and the Rocky Mountain states the lowest. The Plains states seem to be an exception, however. Although there is a large proportion of older residents in this region, their spending and growth were about average.

Medical care spending also varies by condition/disease. The largest source of health care spending is for cardiovascular disease, which accounts for $80 billion (14% of the total spent on medical care). Injuries and the subsequent costs for rehabilitation account for $69 billion, while cancers and genitourinary diseases account for almost $50 billion. The table illustrates medical expenditures by diagnostic category for 1987 (the latest year for which this information was available).

The proposed reform of Medicare should potentially concern employers. Proposed cuts in Medicare spending will undoubtedly cause a shift in the costs of health care to the elderly, to providers and to all health care consumers. At this writing, the picture is anything but clear.

International Comparisons

It is undisputed that the United States leads the world in health care spending. It is also a country that does not guarantee health care to every citizen regardless of the ability to pay. Just about every other industrial nation has a health care system that ensures universal access and coverage and has a uniform payment system and expenditure controls. The United States and South Africa are the only standouts. Other industrialized countries also spend a lower percentage of their GDP on health care, have had more success in controlling health care spending, and require a far smaller share of out-of-pocket spending in total health spending (22.9% in the United States versus 18.4% in Canada, 13.1% in the United Kingdom and 11.1% in Germany). France, Germany and Japan, for example, spend significantly smaller shares of their national income on health care than the United States, and this lower spending has not translated into reduced access to basic health services or to a deterioration in measures of health status.

As in the United States, patients in France, Germany and Japan can choose their own physicians. Unlike the United States, insurance enrollment is compulsory and is provided through a diverse mix of third party payers. A mandated package of health benefits covers a wide range of services. Patients do not pay deductibles, and copayments range from nominal amounts (Germany) to a percent of regulated fees (France and Japan). Workplace-based insurance is financed by employer and employee payroll

TABLE

Medical Expenditures by Diagnostic Category[1]—
United States, 1987
(dollars in billions)[2]

Diagnostic Category	Medical Expenditures	% Total Costs
Cardiovascular	$ 79.6	13.9%
Injury and long-term effects	69.1	12.1
Neoplasm	49.6	8.7
Genitourinary	49.3	8.7
Pregnancy/birth related	39.7	6.9
Respiratory	38.3	6.7
Digestive	35.9	6.3
Musculoskeletal	27.7	4.8
Other circulatory diagnosis	20.2	3.5
Mental health[3]	19.3	3.4
Well care	17.4	3.0
Congenital anomalies	8.7	1.5
Medical misadventure	6.9	1.2
Miscellaneous[4]	110.6	19.3
TOTAL	572.3	100.0

Source: Morbidity and Mortality Weekly Report, 1994.

1. Based on International Classification of Diseases, Ninth Edition, Clinical Modification (ICD-9-CM).

2. Adjusted to December 1993 dollars. Excludes nursing home, dental and insurance claims processing costs.

3. Excludes mental health services without a medical component.

4. Includes carpal tunnel syndrome, endocrine disorders other than diabetes, anemia, conditions that were not clearly attributable to an underlying cause, cataracts and glaucoma.

contributions which reflect the average cost of a larger cross section of the population.

Most importantly, each has imposed direct controls on overall health spending and health care prices. Germany, for example, imposed mandatory global budget limits on spending as an emergency measure to reduce cost pressures, excess service volume and overuse of technology. Compared to the United States, short-term results show that Germany has been more successful in controlling the rate of growth of their health care costs. Whereas the United States expended 14% of its GDP on health care, Germany spent between 8-9% while covering a broad range of health care services for virtually their entire population.

France provides universal coverage via social security and uses a fee-for-service reimbursement system which has resulted in global budgeting to control cost increases. Health care in France consumes 8.6% of the GDP.

Canada has been studied most closely as a model for U.S. health care reform. Canada's publicly funded health care system consists of ten separate provincial plans in which insurance coverage is universal. The provincial governments are the single payers of physicians and hospitals, and they make key decisions on health financing. There are no deductibles or co-payments for covered services. There have been cost problems in Canada, however, and to stay within budget some hospitals and beds have been closed. Shrinking government revenue caused by a recession combined with rising medical costs have clearly jolted the Canadian system, but their cost increases are still less than those of the United States.

In sum, other countries seem to have had better success in controlling their health care costs as a result of a centralization of the cost-control process. The fragmented system in America makes it much harder to effect change.

Peculiarities of the U.S. System

A significant part of the cost problem in the United States stems from the high cost of regulation and microadministration. Estimates of insurance overhead account for nearly one-quarter of total spending. In contrast, administrative costs in other countries total 11% or less. Additionally, in the United States, the philosophy has been that no costs should be spared. The level of unnecessary or inappropriate testing is estimated at $130 billion per year. The United States leads the world in the use of technology. Whereas the utilization rate of CAT and MRI scanners is 44.5 per million population in the United States, in West Germany it is 18.9 per million population and 8.5 per million in Canada. Cardiovascular procedures are performed much more frequently in the United States compared to other nations as well. In most other developed countries, cardiovascular services and elective surgery, in particular, are limited to some extent by the government.

Businesses' Dilemma

Since over 150 million Americans obtain health insurance through their employer, and since businesses spent over $186 billion to provide health benefits to their employees and retirees, the issue is not a trivial one for businesses. What does all this mean for employers? For labor? The answer is simple: Rising health care costs strongly affect the financial condition of all participants in the system.

Health spending by business escalated at more than twice the general inflation rate during the 1980s (+12% compared to 5% for general inflation). Business expenditures for health care have been the most rapidly growing component of employee compensation. Health outlays have more than doubled as a share of total labor compensation (wages, salaries, fringe benefits) from 1970 to 1990. In one decade (1980-1990), employer health care costs as a percentage of total employee wages and salaries increased from 5.8% to 8.5%. Over the same time period, real wages declined slightly. The largest category of health expenditures for business is for employee health insurance.

It is known that health care costs vary widely across businesses. Figure 3 shows the range of costs for health insurance paid by different firms. In 1991, the average combined health care costs per covered worker for employers and employees in wholesale/retail trade were three-fourths of those in manufacturing and two-thirds of those experienced by utilities. Figure 4 shows that other high-cost industries include mining/construction and communications. Health plan costs were at least 20% of payroll in over one-quarter of consumer products firms surveyed, but less than 5% of payroll for one-quarter of firms in technical/professional services. Even within companies in the same industry, costs can vary widely. Among manufacturing companies, 5% had health benefits costs of less than $2,000 per employee while 16% had costs of $5,000 or more. Logically, those firms that have older workers, that cover more retirees, offer a wider range of health benefits and are located in high medical cost areas. Figures 5A and 5B show total 1993 health benefit costs per employee by region.

For those businesses with an aging workforce, rapidly increasing health insurance premiums serve to exacerbate their problems. Increases in coverage costs are a problem for employers with older or less healthy workers as well as those located in high-cost areas. Those with a high percentage of females in the workforce experience higher costs because of the potential for pregnancy and maternity care. Such employers are finding it increasingly difficult to remain competitive while meeting their commitments to employee and retiree benefits. There is concern that businesses will screen future

FIGURE 3

Variation in Average Health Plan Costs, 1991

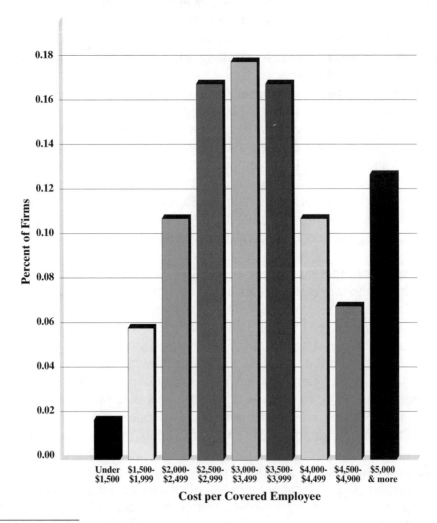

Source: A. Foster Higgins & Co., Inc.

employees on the basis of health status. That is, in an effort to lower health costs, employers might not hire or retain those who have preexisting conditions and/or potentially high health costs (HIV/AIDS, cancer, heart diseases and the like).

An employer's decision to offer health insurance is strongly influenced by its financial condition and the competitive environment. That is, in order

FIGURE 4

Average Health Care Costs by Selected Industries (1991)

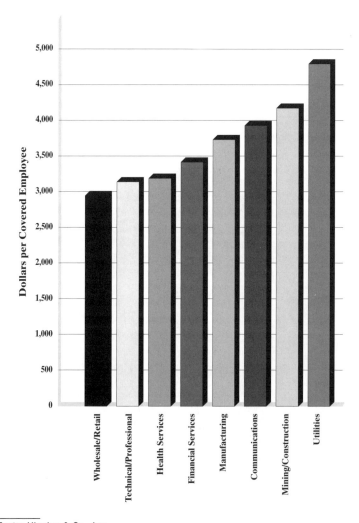

Source: A. Foster Higgins & Co., Inc.

to attract and retain workers, a company may find it necessary to offer a competitive benefits package. While large and medium sized firms continue to offer health benefits to their permanent full-time staff, small businesses often cannot afford to do so. For many small businesses, premiums are generally higher primarily because of the inability to spread risk over a large number of insured; they lack the bargaining power to seek and negotiate

**Total 1991 Health Benefit Cost per Employee by Region
Large Employers**

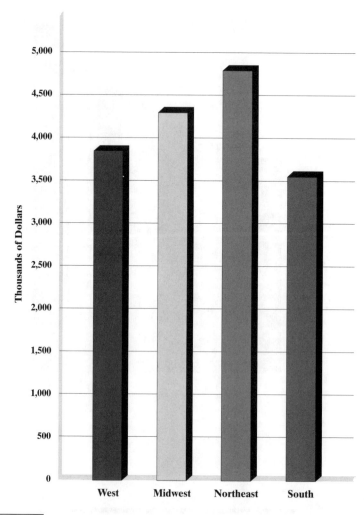

Source: National Survey of Employer-Sponsored Health Plans/1993, A. Foster Higgins & Co., Inc. 1993: New York.

suitable, affordable coverage. Small employers generally experience higher rates of increase in premiums for the same reasons. Small firms are even more vulnerable because one or two employees can threaten their capacity to obtain affordable coverage.

FIGURE 5B

Total 1994 Health Benefit Cost per Employee Region
Small Employers

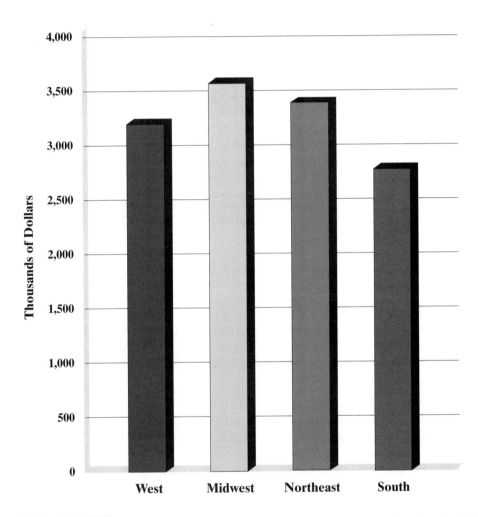

Source: National Survey of Employer-Sponsored Health Plans/1993, A. Foster Higgins & Co., Inc. 1993: New York.

Health Care at the Bargaining Table

Employers have taken action to mitigate the high costs of health care. Some employers have canceled or cut back coverage in response to higher

Health Care Costs and the Effect on Employee Benefits _____ 31

premiums. Most have shifted more of the costs to the employees by raising the deductible employees have to pay out of pocket. Many have decreased their insurance coverage for employees' spouses and dependents, while others do not provide health benefits to part-time or temporary workers. Some have tried to eliminate retiree health benefits, but legal challenges have been mounted successfully in many cases.

Labor's response has been swift and predictable. Labor faces the critical concern of improving, or at least maintaining, the health care provisions of their collective bargaining agreements. Workers are clear that they do not want to be the payer of last resort and are resisting pressure to absorb increased health care costs. When NYNEX attempted to raise employee contributions for health coverage, for example, the members of the Communication Workers union went on strike in protest. NYNEX backed down from its original position. Even before the NYNEX incident, the question of who will pay for the spiraling costs of health care has dominated collective bargaining over the past years. Health care continues to be a major issue in negotiations, according to the Bureau of National Affairs. Increasing employee out-of-pocket costs was the chief reason cited in 90% of labor strikes in the early 1990s.

Light at the End of the Tunnel?

After years of double-digit inflation and increases in premiums, medical inflation and total health benefit costs per employee are beginning to abate. Perhaps employer cost-management efforts are having an effect after all. That is the good news. The bad news is that benefit costs still increased three times the rate of general inflation even though medical care price inflation slowed. This situation leads one to conclude that some of the underlying problems in the financing and delivery of health care remain. This fact should also caution the reader to remain vigilant about cost management and not to become complacent. Each survey is conducted differently, the participating firms in the study sample may differ, the calculations may not be done the same way. Indeed, comparing several surveys of employer-sponsored health plans for 1994, one is immediately struck by the variation in total health benefit costs.

Employers have reacted by having their workers shoulder more of the premium costs. Employer-sponsored health plans are not the open checkbooks that they once were. In fact, the fastest rising component of medical cost increases was increased cost shifting. A more in-depth discussion of employee benefit plans will be offered in Chapter 3. Trends in traditional indemnity medical plans versus managed care plans will be presented and analyzed in regard to cost and design features.

Summary

While employers are taking the cost problem seriously, it should be realized that there is no quick cure for the problems at hand. New services and programs, designed as substitutes for more expensive services and care, have been instituted but, are they truly substitutes or do they add another layer of fat to the already corpulent system? Do they place an increasing burden on the employee to pay for his or her care? This author maintains that the institution of higher deductibles and lower coinsurance, for example, merely transfers formerly paid benefits to the insured consumer and does not contain overall costs.

To address the real cost problem, employers must address the behavior pattern of their employees and, to a large extent, influence provider behavior. Managed care is attempting to control costs in this manner. But, experience suggests that there are no simple solutions to the cost problem. Subsequent chapters will discuss the issue from different angles in an attempt to make some sense out of the crazy patchwork quilt of health care financing and delivery in America.

CHAPTER 3

Employee Benefits: Growth and Options

As the preceding chapters have tried to illustrate, the U.S. health care delivery system is in flux and its configuration is being shaped by a multitude of forces. It is also clear that health care resources are not infinite and that consumers must utilize their dollars in a rational way. Since fringe benefits are often used as a means of attracting and retaining employees, their costs have assumed tremendous importance. The numbers presented sharply indicate that health care benefits are not an incidental cost of doing business. The growth in the scope and cost of benefits has escalated to the point where businesses must be more aware of the economic ramifications of their largesse. There are ways to tailor the benefits package so that costs can be managed better without necessarily sacrificing that which is being offered. This chapter examines benefits options and the means of providing benefits in a cost-efficient manner.

Employment-Based Benefits

Employee benefit plans are most often set up to compensate employees by means of fringe benefits, deferred compensation, retirement/pension plans or a combination thereof. Wayne A. Mehlman's writing[1] on the deductibility and taxation of employee compensation serves as the reference for the following discussion.

In brief, current compensation includes wages and salaries, commissions, bonuses, drawing accounts, vacation pay, gifts, prizes and awards, payments in property and/or services, reimbursement of employee expenses, severance pay and unemployment benefits. These forms of compensation are subject to payroll tax to the employee, although employers may deduct the expenditures *if* they are considered ordinary, necessary and directly connected with their trade or business, reasonable in amount, made for services actually performed, and meet accounting requirements.

Fringe benefits, partially or fully excluded from an employee's gross income, are not subject to payroll taxes and are deductible by the employer, which can only deduct the cost of a fringe benefit and not its value. Typically, fringe benefits include health, dental and accident benefits; disability benefits; group term life insurance coverage; employee death benefits; group legal plans; and qualified tuition reductions, among others.

Deferred compensation plans that meet certain requirements of the Internal Revenue Code permit the employer to deduct contributions while deferring income recognition to the employee until the benefits are actually received by the employee. Included in this definition are pension plans, profit-sharing plans, money purchase plans, target benefit pension plans, Keogh plans, 401(k) plans, individual retirement arrangements, stock bonus plans and employee stock ownership plans. Those plans that do not meet the requirements of the Internal Revenue Code do not receive the same tax advantages as qualified deferred compensation plans; however, they offer greater flexibility.

To be considered a qualified plan, among the requirements are rules concerning who must be covered, how contributions to the plan and benefits under the plan are to be determined, and how much of an employee's interest in the plan is to be invested. Due to the complexity of the laws, a more in-depth discussion can be found elsewhere. Certainly an attorney and tax adviser should be consulted in making any changes to one's benefit plan.

The current tax rules create a significant subsidy for employment-based coverage. The tax exemption of employment-based health insurance is estimated to cost $46 billion in lost federal income tax revenue (1993 dollars). Short-lived efforts to revoke the tax-free status of fringe benefits met with resounding defeat in the early 1990s and, for the moment at least, these benefits enjoy their tax advantage.

---

1. W. A. Mehlman, Special Section on the Deductibility and Taxation of Employee Compensation in *Employee Benefits: Survey Data From Benefit Year 1993,* U.S. Chamber of Commerce.

Although employers initially pay most of the costs for employee health insurance, these costs are largely shifted to the workers in the form of lower real wages and reduced nonmedical benefits. The increase in health costs concomitant with slower growth in productivity and total compensation are the main reasons for the weak growth in workers' real wages and salaries over the past 20 years, according to a Congressional Budget Office report. Its findings show that from 1973 through 1989, employers' contributions to health insurance absorbed more than half of workers' real gains in compensation, even though health insurance represented 5% or less of total compensation. Hence, higher costs for health insurance have had a significant impact on household budgets.

This situation creates an interesting dilemma. Employers have to keep total compensation of workers (wages and benefits) in line with labor productivity. At the same time, workers value the health insurance benefit and are willing to give up some of their income to have it. But, the squeeze has meant that workers' cash wages have barely grown over the past decades, adding tensions between labor and management. Nevertheless, because of rising health care costs, the availability of employer-sponsored health insurance has assumed great importance in choosing a job. Many workers are reluctant to change jobs for fear of losing coverage. The costs of individual health policies, as we all know, are prohibitively expensive. In real terms, what does all this mean? A 1991 study found that workers were willing to give up 82¢ of cash wages for each dollar of health benefits provided by the employer. So, even though rising costs of employer-sponsored health insurance are shifted to the workers (in the form of lower real wages), apparently, the importance of having this benefit is worth the tradeoff.

Growth in Benefits

Table I provides a summary of the growth in employee benefits from 1929 to 1993. In 1929, total benefits were estimated at $1.5 billion, or 3% of the year's $50.4 billion in wages and salaries. At that time, there were no old age, survivors, disability, health insurance or unemployment compensation programs. In fact, the only legally required payments were workers' compensation and governmental employees' retirement. By 1959, benefits totaled $49 billion, or 19% of wages and salaries. Benefits totaled $77 billion (24% of payroll) in 1965 and $691.3 billion in 1985, or 37.7% of payroll.

Total employee benefits exceeded the trillion-dollar mark for the first time in 1990. Benefit costs for all full-time employees were estimated at $1,218.61 billion in 1993, reaching a record 41.3% of payroll. Most re-

TABLE I

Growth of Employee Benefits, 1929 to 1993

	1929	1955	1965	1975	1986	1988	1989	1991	1992	1993
Type of Payment										
Legally required	0.8	3.3	5.3	8.4	11.1	11.6	12.20	12.2	12.1	12.0
Old-Age, Survivors, Disability, and Health Insurance (FICA taxes)	0.0	1.4	2.3	4.6	5.9	6.1	6.5	6.3	6.4	6.3
Unemployment compensation	0.0	0.7	1.0	0.8	1.2	1.0	0.9	0.7	0.9	1.1
Workers' compensation	0.6	0.5	0.7	1.0	1.0	1.6	1.7	1.7	1.8	1.7
Government employees' retirement	0.2	0.5	1.0	1.7	2.8	2.7	2.9	3.2	2.7	2.7
Other	0.0	0.2	0.3	0.3	0.2	0.2	0.2	0.3	0.3	2.0
Agreed upon	0.4	3.6	4.6	7.4	9.7	10.6	11.0	12.7	13.1	14.6
Pensions	0.2	2.2	2.3	3.6	2.8	4.1	4.0	5.1	5.3	5.8
Insurance	0.1	1.1	2.0	3.4	5.6	5.9	6.4	6.7	7.2	7.8
Other	0.1	0.3	0.3	0.4	1.3	0.6	0.6	0.9	0.6	1.0
Rest periods	1.0	3.0	3.1	3.7	3.3	2.9	3.0	2.5	3.1	2.4
Time not worked	0.7	5.9	7.3	9.4	10.2	10.4	10.2	9.9	10.2	9.7
Vacations	0.3	3.0	3.8	4.8	5.2	5.5	5.4	5.2	5.4	5.2
Holidays	0.3	2.0	2.5	3.2	3.1	3.2	3.2	3.1	3.2	2.9
Sick leave	0.1	0.8	0.8	1.2	1.4	1.3	1.2	1.2	1.2	1.2
Other	0.0	0.1	0.2	0.2	0.5	0.4	0.4	0.4	0.4	0.4
Bonuses, profit sharing, etc.	0.1	1.2	1.2	1.1	1.2	1.1	1.1	0.9	0.6	0.6
Total benefit payments (% of wages and salaries)	3.0	17.0	21.5	30.0	35.5	36.7	37.5	38.2	39.1	39.3
Wages and salaries (billions $)	50.5	212.1	363.7	814.7	2,093.	2,431.1	2,573.3	2,816	2,954.8	3,100.8
Total benefit payments (billions $)	1.5	36.1.	78.2	244.4	743.0	813.9	964.98	1,075.7	1,155.3	1,218.6

Source: Estimated by U.S. Chamber of Commerce from U.S. Department of Commerce data and U.S. Chamber of Commerce survey.

sponsible for the continued increase are rising costs of legally required benefits and the continued increase in severance pay and retiree health insurance. The governmental regulations make benefits more costly to employers but do not necessarily increase the benefits available to employees.

FIGURE 1

How the Benefit Dollars Were Spent—1994
Percent of Total

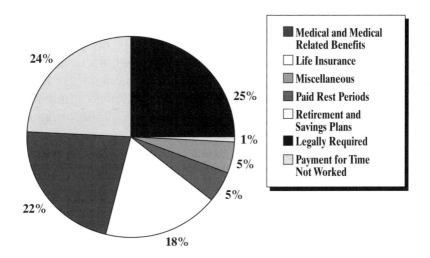

Source: U.S. Chamber of Commerce Employees' Benefits: Survey Data From Benefit Year 1994.

State mandates, too, are pushing up costs. However, in 1994, benefits declined to 40.7% of payroll, almost equaling the 1992 figure of 40.2%.

The 1994 figures compiled by the U.S. Chamber of Commerce say that the steady increase in costs has stopped. In fact, total benefits declined for the first time in the 1990s. Employers' share of medical and medically related costs per employee decreased in 1994. Medically related benefits had increased 14% in 1993 but declined almost half that amount in 1994. The only areas where benefits increased in 1994 were payments for retiree health insurance and payments to defined benefit pension plans.

Figure 1 shows how the benefit dollars were spent in 1994. Leading the list are medical and medical related benefits followed by payment for time not worked. Over one-fifth of the total are legally required benefits, a percentage which has increased steadily over the years.

Employee benefits offered in the 1980s and 1990s evolved over time from plans that addressed the basic needs of workers providing minimum benefits to plans that are much more complex, comprehensive and costly. Employee benefits increased by 8.6% in 1993 in terms of dollars spent per employee per year. In comparison, since payroll costs increased 5.6% in

1993, the increase in benefits represented an increasing percentage of payroll. The largest firms and the older, more established firms spend a greater percentage of payroll on benefits. The top 10% of these firms pay more than 50% of payroll for benefits. Clearly, the cost of medical and medically related benefits contributes to this increase.

It is documented that within industries benefit payments vary widely. Manufacturing firms generally pay more in dollar terms per year per employee for benefits while retailers, textiles, apparel manufacturers and banks tend to have lower benefit levels. Even within industries there are significant variations. Payments in the food, beverage and tobacco industries varied from less than 20% of payroll, for example. Some of the variation in the percent of payroll for benefits is due to differences in pension and profit-sharing payments. But, much of the variation is a product of firm size and age. Regional factors also must be taken into account; the differential between the highest and the lowest cost area regarding the cost of medically related insurance programs is more than 75%!

By region, the East North Central region (Illinois, Indiana, Michigan, Ohio and Wisconsin—the Rust Belt) had highest levels of benefits primarily due to the nature of the companies located there and a high retiree health burden. The Western region had to contend with demographic factors, which influenced benefits packages. Workers in the West tend to be younger and benefits are used to attract more qualified workers. In general, the lowest benefit region is the Southeast (39.1% of payroll) while the East North Central region had the highest level (42.6% of payroll).

What does the future hold? While one or two years do not make a trend, it is of interest to report that benefit costs rose only 0.2% in the first quarter of 1995, the lowest quarterly increase since early 1987. This moderation may reflect a continuing slowdown in the rate of increase in health, workers' compensation and state unemployment insurance costs as well as in employers' payments in retirement funds. Also, the effect of managed care cannot be totally ignored. Time will tell if this dip was an aberration or the beginnings of a turnaround in the costs of employee benefits. However, even though health coverage costs appear to be stabilizing (or decreasing in some cases), employees are still bearing a larger share of the burden of these costs and not reaping the benefits. That is, employees are still paying higher absolute dollar amounts for health coverage in most cases!

Types of Benefits

Although basic hospital-surgical-medical insurance is the most common health benefit provided, many organizations have expanded their benefits package to include dental, vision and prescription drug plans, among other benefits. These benefits can be offered without necessarily squeezing profits. Not surprisingly, there are many ways to offer one or more of these benefits ranging from bare-bones to top-of-the-line coverage. Consideration of the composition of the workforce, finances and philosophy will determine the nature and extent of the benefits package.

Dental Plans

The glut of dentists in the marketplace, the propensity of individuals to ignore preventive dental care, and the costs of root canal and periodontal work are all excellent reasons to implement an employee dental plan. Dental plans, in particular, are prime candidates for some sort of prior authorization or recertification. Since 99% of dental care does not generate enough cost to devastate financially, dental benefit plans, or dental assistance programs, are intended to provide financial assistance rather than catastrophic coverage. In fact, most dental care is for the predictable problems that seldom cost much more than $1,000. For the most part, such plans represent excellent value and are considered a popular benefit.

Dentists, like medical doctors, have an economic incentive to provide more services on a fee-for-service basis. As such, dental plans can do much to monitor quality of care while holding the line on dental expenditures. Recertification of dental treatments may facilitate less costly treatment or the elimination of certain types of recommended care. Indeed, there are many dental treatments covered by standard insurance that are abused, including but not limited to scaling and root work as well as the tremendous inconsistency in the use of X-rays. Services for conditions related to the temporomandibular joint syndrome (TMJ), too, are one of the most rapidly growing areas of abuse. Unnecessary or inappropriate treatment for TMJ costs millions of dollars and may increase health care costs later if they are incorrectly substituted for proper treatment. While dental fraud is difficult to prove, some dental review experts believe that its incidence is significant.

There are four basic categories of dental benefits:
- Preventive and diagnostic services
- Basic restorative services (fillings, extractions, root canal, repair of bridges and partial dentures, treatment of gum and supporting tissue)
- Complex restorative services (inlays, onlays, gold fillings, crowns, bridges, dentures, oral surgery and more major restorative services)
- Orthodontics.

Most dental plans pay 100% of the costs of the preventive and diagnostic services, and require a deductible for basic restorative services. Complex or major restorative services are more costly than basic restorative services and are needed by a smaller portion of the population. A deductible is generally required for these services. Most dental plans include a separate deductible and separate copay for coverage of orthodontic benefits. Usually, there is a lifetime maximum of some dollar amount per child treated.

Any dental plan should have an eligibility and payment structure set up to take into account the effects of projected high utilization. As a rule, the more educated the work population and the more women and children included, the greater the use of dental benefits. Regional variation in utilization must be considered. Curettage and root planing procedures, for example, take place 400-500 times more frequently in New York City than anywhere else in the country.

As a rule of thumb, both the employee and employer should contribute to the dental plan, and the cost should be dependent on whether just the employee is covered or if dependents are included.

Whichever plan one decides on, the following should be considered seriously:

- Strongly encourage alternate, less costly treatment. There are options in dentistry; is the particular service or treatment the most appropriate and cost-effective?
- Do not pay 100% of usual and customary charges. As claims costs increase, the fee schedule approach is much more attractive than paying a fixed percentage of a dentist's usual fee. No plan should pay charges in excess of usual and customary.
- Don't cover dental services in a medical plan.
- Be sure to institute deductibles and copayments.
- Institute an annual maximum for the plan.
- Review claims and seriously consider instituting prospective certification of costly services.
- Consider contracting with a managed dental plan.

What about managed dental plans? The managed dental care industry, while growing annually, is still in the formative stages of development. Primarily because half of all dental fees are paid for out of pocket, there has not been as much pressure for managed dental care. This situation may be changing.

Briefly, managed dental care is generally characterized by the following:

- A dental plan receives a premium from a group or individual as prepayment for a specific set of benefits.
- The dental plan arranges for the benefits to be delivered through a network of providers.
- The network providers are screened for competence and agree to fol-

low some type of quality measures, which may include chart audits or submission of utilization data.

- Network providers are compensated by the dental plan either under a capitation system or by some type of discounted fee schedule.

But, does managed dental care make sense for your organization? Unlike medicine, data on the extent of dental benefits in general and the growth of managed dental plans in particular are sketchy. The National Association of Dental Plans, in collaboration with InterStudy, found that the growth rate for dental HMOs is significant: a 16% annual growth rate. However, key issues should be addressed by potential clients. First, it is important to quantify the extent of unnecessary/inappropriate care. Second, how should one define *dental quality*? Third, what type of savings can one expect? Premiums for dental HMOs remain significantly below their indemnity competitors. Fourth, what are the qualifications of the network dentists?

Since managed care dentistry is still very much of a cottage industry, especially compared to medicine, it is harder to make a recommendation. Each organization will have to assess its dental costs to determine whether managed dental care makes sense. Some experts have questioned the economic wisdom of the concept: Since dental claims involve comparatively small amounts of money, it may not be worth the investment of time and money to set up.

Another option is to self-fund a dental plan. What one has to do first, however, is to estimate how much the plan will cost; if the cost is too high, the plan can be redesigned to include fewer benefits. Self-funded dental plans can offer significant advantages over insured plans in terms of flexibility and better cost management.

Vision Plans

Many plans do not provide a nonmedical vision care benefit even though vision benefits are generally regarded as an inexpensive means of enhancing an employee benefits program. Utilization rates and costs are predictable and not likely to cause catastrophic risks. The popularity of this benefit is best illustrated by its growth. By the mid-1990s, the percentage of employers offering this benefit was over 80%.

Vision care coverage refers to a separate plan covering medical treatment relating to eye care. Ophthalmologists, optometrists or opticians can render care. Since seven of every ten working adults wear some form of corrective lenses, and since the cost of eye wear has escalated, it is not surprising that a vision plan is extremely popular with employees. Vision plans tend to focus on providing frames, lenses and contacts in addition to the annual eye exam.

Vision plans can help address and correct potentially costly and devastating eye problems in the future. Many adults and children do not receive vision examinations on a routine basis and, as such, run the risk of developing serious and potentially costly eye problems. For example, in its early stages, glaucoma can be detected and treated; left untreated, the individual runs the risk of blindness.

There are several ways of implementing an eye care benefit. A reimbursement indemnity plan combined with a provider network can be an excellent cost-containment approach. There are managed vision groups that offer vision care at discounted rates. Optometrists and ophthalmologists employed by a managed care organization would provide all eye care. In such an integrated system, the optometrist acts as the eye care gatekeeper and can quickly refer a patient when there is a need for more specialized care. Typically, an employee would be entitled to an annual eye exam and glasses/contacts if needed. There should be a maximum amount allowed for frames, and anything above that maximum would be paid for out of pocket.

Prescription Drug Plans

Prescription drugs potentially represent the greatest out-of-pocket expense for Americans, especially the older members of society. Approximately 70% of medications are ordered for long-term use, and the costs associated with this are not insignificant. The price of prescription drugs has been rising sharply: From 1980 to 1990, expenditures for prescription drugs grew at an average annual rate of 9%. By 1990, total drug expenditures totaled $48.5 billion and, by 1993, reached an estimated $58 billion. It is estimated that drug costs will be $91 billion by the year 2000. Clearly, employers realize that there is a need to focus on managing prescription drug expenditures, including a focus on employee usage and provider practices.

The growing proportion of total medical costs attributed to prescription drug benefits reflects not only price increases but also changing utilization rates. There is a broader use of prescription drugs by individuals of all ages. One survey found that the average number of prescriptions filled annually was 4.4. Concomitantly, the prices of the top selling brand-name prescription drugs increased more than 1½ times faster than the general rate of inflation from 1993 to 1994. Table II shows the costs of common prescription drugs as well as the cumulative price changes from 1989 to 1994. The results are startling.

For years, the consumer was fairly insensitive to rising costs. But, with the rapid increases in common prescription drugs, and the psychological shift of focus regarding health care costs, the behavior of the consumer and those paying the bills is changing. There has been a concerted effort to rein in phar-

TABLE II

Top Selling Brand-Name Prescription Drugs, 1994

BRAND NAME	MEDICAL USE	EXPENDITURES (in millions)	CUMULATIVE PRICE CHANGE 1984-1994 (%)
PROZAC	Depression	$ 72.270	58.0%
ZANTAC	Ulcer	59.827	38.0
TAGAMET	Ulcer	43.155	52.5
MEVACOR	Cholesterol	34.116	27.8
PROCARDIA XL	Blood Pressure	26.140	58.4
PREMARIN	Estrogen	25.935	85.3
PRILOSEC	Ulcer	20.546	21.1
SELDANE	Antihistamine	20.435	63.0
ANGMENTIN	Antibiotic	19.678	63.1
CARDIZEM CD	Angina	18.112	48.9

Source: Families USA, 1995. PRIME Institute, University of Minnesota.

maceutical costs and to be more aware of options. One of the easiest and earliest actions has been to have prescriptions filled under the generic drug name. It is no secret that brand-name drugs cost more than their generic equivalents which, according to the Food and Drug Administration, offer the same therapeutic benefits.

While costs have provided the impetus for action, there is also a medical rationale to make the system more efficient. For the most part, the system of prescribing, dispensing and monitoring the use of prescription drugs has largely been uncoordinated and poorly managed. Patients are often treated by several physicians who may not know what the others are, or are not, prescribing. Some patients may be overprescribed while others are underprescribed. What was needed was a system which would operate in an economically efficient manner as well as assist patients in adhering to proper drug therapy.

Not surprisingly, within the last few years, the managed care concept has been applied to prescription drugs. Managed care tries to ensure that the patient will get the most beneficial and cost-effective medication regardless of manufacturer. Key components include the ability to check a patient's medical and prescription drug histories and coordinate the prescription drug treatment. The pharmacy benefit manager has emerged as a key person to monitor drug utilization as well as drug costs. Pharmacy benefit management companies are compiling huge databases and using the information to manage disease by focusing on:

- Appropriate utilization
- Patient education
- Network coordination and management
- Quality assurance and outcomes measurement.

One possible conflict of interest comes to mind, however. While the Food and Drug Administration has clear standards for pharmaceutical manufacturers with regard to drug promotion, there is no regulation of pharmacy benefit management companies (usually owned or controlled by large pharmaceutical companies), giving rise to the question of objectivity and unbiased drug therapy recommendations.

There are many different prescription drug plans, and each employer should consider all options and then select the plan or program that will best serve its needs. The aim should be to develop a program that provides access to prescription drugs, eliminates unnecessary and inappropriate compliance, and improves a patient's health status.

A well-designed plan can help contain costs. Prescription drug vendors offer an array of drug benefit arrangements from simple volume discounts to complex online and retrospective review programs designed to improve clinical outcomes of drug therapy. Some of the plan options include prescription card service and mail-order drug programs. Both offer discounts as a means of containing prescription drug costs. Drug card programs have the advantage of having comprehensive patient information, which can help eliminate contraindications based on the individual's medical history, as well as simplify billing. Drug cards, however, have sometimes been associated with excess and inappropriate use by nonplan members. Card programs may also increase the number of drug claims paid by the employer.

Mail-order plans are relatively easy to implement and cost-effective (potential savings can be generated through volume purchasing and using lower cost generic substitutes). A mail-order program's centralized administration and utilization review can increase efficiency. But, mail-order programs may cause higher costs and excessive distribution if plans are not well designed and administered.

Whichever type of plan is selected, it should offer a variety of cost-management techniques such as utilization review, review for fraud and abuse, a cap on covered expenses and a separate deductible. The growing use of drug therapy in treating a wider range of medical conditions makes it imperative that employers seek cost-effective ways to modify prescription drug benefits. Some employers have been more successful than others in achieving cost savings. Clearly, vendor selection and plan design are critical factors influencing cost. But, the potential for savings is great, especially with the growing competition among drug plan vendors. Deeper discounts are being offered along with more effective clinical review.

Work and Family Benefits

As lifestyles become more complex, employees' needs change, and employers have become responsive to these changing needs. There is a growing need for *work family benefits:* unpaid personal leave of absence, dependent care spending accounts, coverage or well-baby care, personal days, gradual return to work, and the like. Many employers report that they feel that they "need" to offer many of these options in order to compete in the labor market and to add to the perception that the company is "a good place to work for." Whether these type of benefits are cost-effective has not been empirically shown; however, it makes sense to assume that psychologically they are well worth it.

A Hewitt Associates survey on work and family benefits found that employers are offering more of these benefits to meet the demands of their employees' family life. Eighty-four percent of employers offer some kind of care assistance; most prevalent are dependent care spending accounts, and resource and referral services. Much of the interest and establishment of these programs stems from the Family and Medical Leave Act of 1993, which required employers to provide 12 weeks of unpaid family and medical leave for the birth/adoption of a child or for the serious illness of a family member.

Prepaid Legal Plans

While not as prevalent as the above benefit options, prepaid legal care is being offered by more employers as a "hot" employee benefit. Prepaid legal services operate much the same way as health maintenance organizations for medical care. Employees would pay a flat fee—usually $10-$20 a month—and would be able to use the services of a network of lawyers to handle house closing, drafting of wills, divorce, and the like. Excluded are defense against criminal charges. Is prepaid legal cost-effective? An employer is not offering this as a benefit to save money. It is a nice perk.

Plan Design

Options

The benefits discussed above represent the most frequently offered benefits by employers. The type of benefit plan offered is strongly influenced by employer size, location, industry type and collective bargaining agreements. Funding methods also play an important part in determining the scope of benefits offered as well as benefit cost. That is, the key elements of plan design are the scope of benefits covered, the level to which the plan will reimburse employees for covered expenses, and the amount of the deductible and coinsurance.

By the early 1990s, traditional indemnity medical plans were the most common type of employer-sponsored health insurance plan. The majority of such plans embody a comprehensive major medical plan in which reimbursement for health services is subject to both a deductible and coinsurance. The average deductible in 1994 was $231, with regional differences evident: $326 in the West to $186 in the Midwest. Most employers cap a family's deductible either through a predetermined annual amount (usually $500 or more per family) or by limiting the number of family members required to meet the annual deductible. Employers also limit their employees' maximum annual out-of-pocket liability (average set at $1,600). The typical employee co-insurance is 20% of covered health care expenses. Almost all indemnity plans include some form of utilization management/cost management such as precertification of hospital admissions, or case management or quality assessment.

However, as the chapter on managed care will show, the percentage of employees enrolled in traditional indemnity plans is rapidly falling. Most employers now offer options or choices, and those health plans which combine elements of traditional indemnity coverage with those of managed care network plans (combination plans) are becoming most prevalent. These plans offer enrollees access to HMO-like benefits within a managed care network along with some level of indemnity coverage for care received outside the network.

As the delivery and financing of employee benefits undergo a transformation, employers are aware that it is very difficult to meet all employees' needs with a single benefits package. Offering a choice in benefits makes it more likely that employers and employees will get the maximum value from their benefit dollars. Redesign of benefits packages to be more responsive to the needs of the employee, ensuring flexibility in design, has become a key factor in the benefits field. The following is a brief discussion of the concept.

Flexible Benefit Plans

The array of benefit possibilities raises basic issues of employer philosophy. Each employer must decide how it wishes to modify its compensation/benefits package to enable employees to meet their needs more effectively. *Flexible compensation* refers to a means of delivering benefits to employees under which each individual has some choice as to the form of all or a portion of benefits which will best meet personal needs.

The concept of flexible benefit plans was codified under Section 125 of the Internal Revenue Code, which offered employers a choice between permissible taxable benefits and nontaxable health and welfare benefits such as life and health insurance, vacation pay, retirement plans and child care. The employee can then determine how his or her benefit dollars will be allocated for each type of benefit from the total amount promised by the employer. Flexibility allows employees to trade benefits that they do not need for those that they want, at no additional cost to the employer. Most flexible benefit plans have a core set of benefits that every employee gets; employees then tailor the rest of the benefits and compensation package to meet their own specific circumstances.

The typical full flexible benefit plan includes core benefits of medical, life insurance, short- and long-term disability, 401(k) plan and vacation/holiday benefits. Not surprisingly, benefit and personnel practices vary among different industries, regions and organization sizes. Overall, flexible benefit plans are offered by 81% of employers, although these plans are rarely found in organizations with fewer than 500 employees.

What do employees think about employee benefits? Which benefits are important to them? A 1995 Colonial Life and Accident Insurance company survey polled respondents to rank the importance of selected employee health benefits. As Figure 2 shows, major medical benefits ranked the highest in importance followed by prescription drugs and cancer coverage. Another 1995 survey conducted by Hewitt Associates found that the most prevalent area of benefit flexibility was the provision of pretax premiums and spending accounts followed by alternative work arrangements (flextime, compressed workweeks, job sharing and telecommuting). Long-term care insurance is being considered by many employers to meet the growing needs/fears of an aging workforce.

Different findings from different surveys reflect that employees have different needs and would like their benefits package to reflect these differences. Also, needs change over time, and employees prefer tailoring their benefits to their changing needs. Employers have responded by incorporating choice in the form of flexible benefit plans.

Many flexible benefit programs include *flexible spending accounts (FSAs)*, which give employees a choice between taxable cash and nontaxable compensation in the form of payment or reimbursement of eligible, tax-favored welfare benefits. FSAs can be funded through salary reduction, employer contribution, or a combination of both. Employees can purchase

FIGURE 2

How Working Americans Ranked the Importance of Employer-Sponsored Health Care Benefits

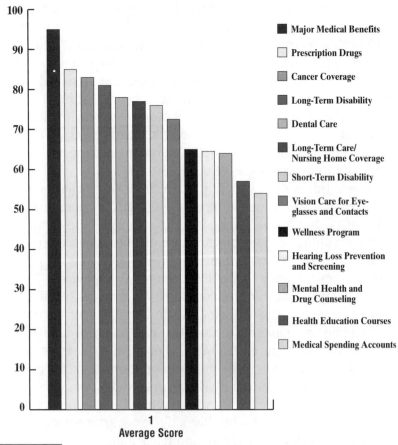

Source: Colonial Life and Accident Insurance Company, 1995 survey.

additional benefits, pay health insurance deductibles and copayments, or pay for child-care benefits with the money in their FSAs or through payroll deductions. Many flexible benefit programs provide employees with a specific amount of dollars or credits that they can use to purchase benefits or convert to take-home pay. Vacation trading is an attractive option as well. Dental options are included under most flexible benefit plans as are life insurance choices. Fewer than one-third of employers with such plans offer short-term disability or sick leave options, primarily because the potential for adverse selections can be high.

Employers have started to offer less traditional benefits to employees who would be able to buy them through payroll deductions or by choosing them as part of a flexible benefit plan. Group auto insurance is one of the latest offerings as are homeowners insurance, long-term care insurance, financial planning services and supplemental disability insurance. While the percentage of employers offering some of these benefits is small (<15%), interest is growing. These policies sound appealing to employees and are easily offered in any flexible benefit plan.

The cornerstone of many flexible benefit plans is a 401(k) plan with elective contributions. In fact, a 401(k) plan is a low-cost way to try flexibility without committing to a full-scale program. These plans are named after the section of the Internal Revenue Code that authorized them in 1978. They enable employees to make pretax contributions by salary reduction agreements structured within the format of a cash or deferred plan, thus reducing the employee's tax bracket. The plan is popular because it permits employees to save for retirement on a pretax basis and, in many cases, employers match employee contributions.

Logically, a flexible benefit program with numerous options is more complex to administer. In a flexible program all participants must be enrolled annually, and some information must be personalized. Administratively, the system must be able to track options selected by employees. There are many decisions that must be agreed upon, including (1) the frequency of allowable payments from an FSA, (2) the handling of credits and (3) core benefits and option prices when an employee's pay changes during the year. Fortunately, there are excellent computer software programs available.

Before setting up a flexible benefit plan, it is important to do your homework. Among other things:

- Review your current package, including benefit plan record-keeping.
- Assess the personnel and their qualifications as applied to the handling of the existing plan.
- Identify changes needed to administer the proposed program.
- Identify procedures that should be computerized.
- Determine if the system should be developed internally or if a vendor should be hired.
- Involve employees by surveying their needs and preferences, educating them about flexibility, and gaining their commitment and appreciation.
- Assess the staff required to administer the proposed plan.
- Assess the ability of the current communications program to meet the needs of proposed changes.

- Be sure that management makes the final decision on the scope and extent of the flexible benefit program.
- Evaluate and monitor the plan to see if it is achieving its objectives.

Data from various studies uniformly show that flexible benefit programs are quite popular with employers and employees. Over 18 million Americans have taken advantage of this tax-advantaged vehicle. A 1994 Gallup Poll found that employees prefer having a choice. Most flex programs, for example, provide a choice of medical plans. Although the traditional indemnity plan is the most common type of medical plan offered under flexible plans, employers rely heavily on managed care plans as well. Of note, although flexible benefit plan sponsors report success in controlling health care costs under this plan design, these companies had a higher average 1993 total health cost ($3,918) than employers without a flexible plan ($5,587). One possible explanation is that employers with higher-than-average costs are more likely to implement a flexible benefit plan. Overall, almost half of employers said that their flexible benefit program helped reduce plan costs because their employees elected more cost-effective medical plan options.

In summary, flexible benefit plans are popular among employers and employees alike. The employer can be benevolent by giving employees a choice of benefits while helping to control costs. While most companies follow the Department of Labor guidelines on basic features of a good 401(k) plan, there is plenty of room for discretion. Employees benefit by individualizing their compensation package to fashion a personal financial program. They can trade benefits that they do not need for ones that they want at no additional cost to the employer.

The Self-Funding Option

In an effort to try to reduce the expenses against an experienced plan, many employers have opted to self-insure. *Self-funding, self-insurance* or *self-administration plans* refer to the provision of health benefits without involving an intermediate insurance carrier. A fully noninsured or *self-insured plan* is one in which the insurance company or service plan collects no premiums and assumes no risk. The employer is fully responsible for all costs. In a sense, the employer is acting as an insurance company—paying no claims with the money ordinarily earmarked for premiums. By retaining funds until claims become due, a company that is self-insured realizes substantial cash flow advantages and the potential of substantial dollar savings. The opportunity to gain enhanced investment income or reserves formerly held by the insurance carrier is there.

Self-insurance has grown dramatically over the past five years, primarily because of ever-increasing medical care costs and an increased awareness of the effectiveness of self-insurance. Those who decide to self-insure do so because they have determined that they can save money by assuming the risk with the additional advantage of total control over the design, funding and administration of the plan. There is often more control over the funds and a better control of provider abuse if an organization self-funds.

The election of self-insurance implies that the employer agrees to assume greater fiduciary and legal responsibilities. The employer or trust fund agrees to pay claims up to a prearranged limit beyond which they would purchase insurance coverage to protect against unpredictable or catastrophic losses (partial self-insurance). It is of paramount importance to operate with sufficient reserves; proper claims accounting is a must. Careful cash management is essential to the self-funding process, since claims and expenses are paid for out of the sum of money received from contributions. Legal requirements delineate the requirements for those who choose to self-insure.

To help determine the feasibility of self-funded insurance, several questions should be considered seriously:

- Does the organization have a large enough number of employees/ members to allow for the necessary spread of risk?
- What has been the organization's claims experience?
- Is there high claim frequency and low claim severity?
- Can the organization's administration handle all aspects of self-insurance?
- Does the organization have suitable cash flow to borrow money to cover aggregate claims throughout the year?

Savings are likely to be realized in several ways: By maintaining a reserve, self-funded plans accumulate their own interest on deposits held to pay claims; by eliminating state premium or franchise taxes by paying for claims only after they have been incurred; by not paying retention charges to an insurance company. Self-funded plans are regulated by the Employee Retirement Income Security Act (ERISA) and, as such, are exempt from state jurisdiction in the regulation of insurance.

To help determine whether self-funding is feasible, the following questions should be addressed:

- How much will be needed to pay for claims?
- How much money in reserve is needed?
- What is the extent of catastrophic losses?
- How will the investments be handled?
- How will the collections be handled?
- How much will it cost to administer the plan?
- How will the plan be audited to check abuses?

Most self-insured employers and trust funds do not have their own system of processing claims. Many have a third party administrator (TPA) take care of this task. Others elect an administrative services only (ASO) with an insurance carrier. To assess the flexibility of the TPA or ASO, the following should be considered:

- Can the organization handle present as well as future needs?
- Can its system handle several different plans?
- How much experience has the organization had in handling group health claims?
- Is the organization approved by a stop-loss (insurance) company?
- Is the fee a fixed amount per employee? What services are included in the fee?
- What is the organization's financial stability?
- Does the organization implement cost-management measures?
- How will the organization track claims, gather and analyze data, and issue reports?

If an employer decides to handle the claims process in-house, the size of the staff must be considered since the number of personnel will depend upon the individual organization's size, needs and ability to process claims quickly and efficiently. A strong administrator is needed to assure that the claims paying process and other administrative functions run smoothly. Any organization thinking of processing its own claims must have a thorough grasp of the realities of the situation. One of the disincentives to processing health care claims in-house is that all complaints will come directly to the employer.

Regardless of who is processing the claims, it is essential to have claims audited by an outside consultant. Also, strict confidentiality and nondisclosure of information to those inside and outside the organization must be maintained.

In summary, opting for self-insurance most probably will result in elimination of, or a substantial reduction in, premium taxes, insurance company retention, recovery of reserves and enhanced investment income. Self-funding also provides the opportunity to reduce unnecessary treatment and provider charges. It provides a high degree of flexibility in benefits schedules. However, there is no assurance of continued savings without implementation of cost-containment programs. Self-insurance cannot work in a vacuum. Such plans must promote the use of the most cost-efficient type of care.

Summary

The complexity of providing employee benefits has evolved over the decades to a point where both employers and employees have numerous options to consider. While this chapter provided a brief overview of the field, it should have made clear that providing employee benefits is not an incidental cost of doing business. Under the circumstances, it is important that each individual organization custom design its program to meet its own needs. Flexibility is a key component for any system. Consideration of demographics of the workforce, financial considerations, cooperation between management and labor, each contributes to and determine the nature and extent of an employee benefits package.

Cost-containment mechanisms can and should be implemented regardless of the size of the company. The growth in the cost of benefits and the percent of payroll attributed to benefits are too large to ignore.

CHAPTER 4

The Age of Managed Care

The cornerstone of most benefit plans had been the traditional indemnity plan, which was the major determinant of overall rising benefit costs. The recent upheavals in health care delivery and financing, however, have shifted the focus away from indemnity plans to managed care. The data clearly show that the conventional models of health insurance, those with no constraints on choice of providers or utilization controls, are becoming a thing of the past. The timing was right for managed care to proliferate, and it filled a void. But, is it the answer to the health care cost crisis? The jury is still out.

Managed care, the newest watchword of cost containment, has become synonymous with enrollment in a health maintenance organization (HMO), preferred provider organization (PPO) or a review program managed by a third party. The basic objective is to manage utilization and price by controlling the type, level and frequency of treatment and by restricting the level of reimbursement for services. A fundamental feature is to direct patients to a closed panel of providers who have agreed to practice less costly, more efficient medicine, as dictated by the managed care organization. Managed care plans gain leverage in negotiating prices and utilization by concentrating patients among few providers.

According to Enthoven, the chief promulgator of managed competition, the new system's objective is to obtain maximal value for consumers and employers by using rules for competition derived from microeconomic principles. Organizations compete in terms of price and quality, using market forces to develop efficient delivery systems; those that develop the most efficient delivery systems by improving quality, cutting costs and satisfying patients will thrive, theoretically.

With this new system of delivery has come a new set of terms such as *integrated delivery systems,* which provide alternatives to the traditional fee-for-service indemnity health plans; *managed indemnity plans,* in which the insurer relies on utilization controls to manage the practices of providers that it reimburses; and *case management,* in which usually a nurse is responsible for coordinating the care for high-risk patients with expensive conditions (e.g., cancers, neonatal care, acquired immunodeficiency syndrome).

Managed care has evolved considerably from the prototype HMO developed by Kaiser Permanente, the nation's oldest and largest HMO. In the early 1970s, HMOs were touted as effective alternatives for the control of health care costs. The HMO Act of 1973 established regulations and qualifications standards for HMOs and, since then, their growth has been steady and impressive, particularly in the 1980s and 1990s.

Managed care arrangements continue to undergo dynamic changes as enrollment expands and patient/consumer demands change. The mechanisms designed to control costs and use of services, however, are basically the same although plans vary widely on how providers are selected, the method of reimbursement, the effectiveness of utilization management, and the extent of enrollee and provider incentives.

Provider Selection and Reimbursement

Most HMOs rely on a physician *gatekeeper,* usually a family practitioner, who coordinates care and is supposed to guard against excessive use of the health care system without denying necessary treatment. Cost reduction is attempted by negotiating lower prices for health services or providing hospitals and physicians with financial incentives to provide fewer services. By shifting some financial risk to providers, it is thought that extensive use of referrals and expensive services will be discouraged.

By channeling enrollees to a limited number of providers, the HMO has leverage in price negotiations and provides more control over utilization. Some plans employ rigorous selection criteria to choose the most cost-effective providers, but most plans select providers that meet minimum professional standards and are willing to contract with the plan. Some managed care plans also contract exclusively with groups of physicians rather than physicians in individual practices. Research has shown that physicians in multispecialty group practices have lower hospital admission rates than physicians in individual practice plans regardless of whether the patient is in an indemnity plan or a managed care plan.

Some plans accept *any willing provider,* which means that any licensed provider willing to agree to reimbursement and utilization control mechanisms can join. Board certification is not a requirement. Before contracting with any plan, one should query how the plan credentials its providers.

Many plans prepay providers (using a capitation rate), while others have physicians on salary. With prepayment, the provider is responsible for rendering care but does not receive a payment for each service, which places the risk of costly services on the provider but rewards him or her if less costly care is provided. Indeed, prepayment has been associated with lower levels of utilization, but the employer usually does not benefit from this situation. It is the provider who benefits. To achieve cost savings, the employer must negotiate a capitation rate lower than the average cost would have been if paid for by fee for service.

Types of HMOs

The early HMOs employed physicians (staff models) whose compensation would not be directly related to the level of services provided. Over time, HMOs evolved into *individual practice associations (IPAs)*. IPAs have an administrative and management group that contracts with independent physicians and other providers. The HMO collects premiums and pays the providers according to a schedule based primarily on actual utilization. IPA doctors see patients (HMO enrollees and others) in their own offices. In an IPA arrangement, physicians are reimbursed primarily on a fee-for-service basis so that their compensation tends to increase if they provide more care.

In a group model HMO, physicians are partners in a group practice and their compensation is directly dependent on the financial success of the HMO. Under this model, there is a strong incentive to provide cost-effective treatment and to curtail unnecessary services.

While employers have gravitated to the managed care approach to health care delivery and financing, their employees made it quite clear that they want freedom to choose their own provider. Indeed, it is this issue that proved to be most contentious. The doctor-patient relationship is an important component in the American psyche and most individuals rebelled at the thought that they would not be able to continue seeing their own private doctor. The perceived imposition of creating a business relationship between doctor and patient angered most.

As a direct result of consumer displeasure, a new variation on the HMO evolved: the open-ended HMO or *point-of-service (POS)* HMO. Under many typical plans, an employer would offer employees the choice of joining an HMO and the employee would have to select a physician from a preset list of providers. Many employees were reluctant to join an HMO which did not offer freedom of choice. Consumers wanted the right to choose their own doctor; by design, managed care constrained choice by contracting with specific providers. If one's personal physician was not a contractor, one had to change providers to receive full reimbursement. So, in response to the loud and negative reaction to such restrictions, many employers established a POS option that permits employees to receive care from the provider of their choice by paying additional out-of-pocket costs. POS plans are more costly than closed-ended plans, but employers viewed the compromise as worthwhile.

Another hybrid managed care product, which is an indemnity-based alternative, is being marketed: *exclusive provider organization (EPO)*. An EPO requires enrollees to use the network providers exclusively, but the EPO has more choice of providers than most HMOs because the former's provider network size tends to be more generous than the latter's. If the enrollee seeks care out of the network, however, they are usually not reimbursed for costs incurred.

EPOs, like HMOs, utilize gatekeepers and rely on negotiated fees and indemnity-based payments. In contrast, many HMOs rely on capitation. EPOs' other features include flexible benefit design, flexible funding, claim-for-service indemnity payment and experience rating. EPOs can compete with HMOs without having to meet strenuous HMO licensing requirements. Many employers will use an EPO for specialized services such as obstetrics, cardiac care, organ transplants, cancer care and psychiatric care.

Who's buying EPOs? EPOs often do best in mature managed care markets where employers have experienced the alternatives. Small employers, too, would do well to consider an EPO. The compact size of the EPO network can be a selling point to small employers.

Preferred Provider Organizations

In addition to the HMO, a network of providers called *preferred provider organizations (PPOs)* emerged. Frustration led many employers to contract with providers who agreed to provide services at a discounted rate. These PPOs began to proliferate in the 1980s. Under the PPO concept, providers offered negotiated discounts from normal fees to participants who elected to use their services in exchange for increased volume of patients and timeliness of payment. Discounts generally range between 15-20% below billed charges, but vary by type of provider, geographic location and markup over cost.

As with an HMO, an essential element of a successful PPO is the ability to identify efficient health care providers who provide quality care at reasonable cost. While the cost potential of PPOs results from the negotiated arrangement, there is a persistent concern that the original fee might have been inflated to compensate for the discount. While doctors agree to reduce fees charged for services, many make up for the loss by increasing volume. That is, a PPO doctor can ask that the patient come back more often or can order more lab tests; such actions clearly minimize cost-effectiveness. Another problem is the lack of uniform standards for quality under this arrangement. Unlike HMOs, PPOs are unregulated.

Ironically, as PPOs evolved during the 1980s, they became more like HMOs. In some cases the only differences between HMOs and some PPOs were that employees had to make an exclusive one-year commitment to enroll in an HMO and that providers in PPOs shared less of the risk.

Attentive to the need to manage costs, yet do so by offering health benefit programs that employees find attractive, many employers are offering plan combinations, which enable the employer to provide a full range of health care benefits while allowing for employee freedom of choice. A common plan of this sort would consist of an HMO, a PPO and a modified indemnity plan. Very few employers offer only a HMO plan or only an indemnity plan, for example. Of course, the employer can structure the overall program to encourage participation in managed care options by providing financial incentives.

Growth and Consolidation of Managed Care Plans

Managed care has emerged as the primary vehicle for cost control in the United States. By the end of 1994, managed care served over 56 million people, and is growing geometrically. In 1995, the number of commercial HMOs, for example, rose over 7% and nationwide enrollment increased 10%. The annual compounded growth of leading HMOs exceeded 30% in the early 1990s, and the growth rate for the rest of the decade appears to be equally strong, particularly if managed care is mandated for Medicare and Medicaid recipients. Overall, IPAs represent 65% of all HMOs and clearly dominate the market at this point in time. In contrast, PPOs grew only 3%.

The penetration of managed care in markets that had traditionally been resistant has been impressive. The arrival of the big national players in the New York metropolitan market, for example, appears to have opened up a previously skeptical market. From 1992 to 1995, there was almost a 10% increase in managed care contracts in the New York City area compared to a 4.8% increase nationwide.

Within the managed care industry there has been much turmoil. The mid-1990s witnessed a flurry of mergers and acquisitions. In 1994 alone, publicly traded HMOs completed 13 acquisitions totaling over $4 billion. Ironically, as the market is expanding and growing, the number of players is being constricted; but, merger mania does not appear to be over yet. There were a record 178 transactions that were publicly announced during the third quarter of 1995 alone, for example. Four of the ten largest HMOs, for example, have cash and investments exceeding $1 billion. The *Wall Street Journal* has predicted that by 1996, there will be a handful of companies competing for a potential $200 billion market, which would create a tremendous concentration of market power in the hands of a few organizations.

While the market has been consolidating horizontally, hospitals, physicians and insurers have also been expanding vertically by merging and acquiring each other. Adding to the already extensive listing of alphabet soup acronyms, the *physician-hospital organization (PHO)* has been added to the managed care lexicon. These alliances are being formed to help health care providers attain market share, improve bargaining power and reduce administrative costs. PHOs align hospitals and physicians in order to maintain and expand joint market share through joint contracting. PHOs sell their services to managed care organizations or directly to employers.

Since two competitors (hospitals and physicians) are forming a single entity for business purposes, in a sense forming a joint venture, antitrust issues must be assessed. The concept is so new that legal positions have not been formalized. At the moment, too, these entities are unregulated, unlike HMOs.

What is clear is that in order to succeed, the PHO would need sufficient size to penetrate a market; a small PHO probably would not be able to last in a competitive field. If, however, the PHO is properly organized, capitalized and administered, it could potentially be effective. In one sense, PHOs represent the beginnings of an *integrated delivery system (IDS),* another newcomer to the field.

The formation of vertically integrated networks, such as IDSs, is taking place as managed care plans increase their penetration and competitive markets become more mature. IDSs differ from PHOs in several ways: PHOs are formed primarily to win managed care contracts. IDSs use clinically driven models (outcomes research, practice guidelines) to fuel product selection. Clinical integration determines where care is delivered within the system and directs patients to specific physicians and clinics rather than duplicating services at a number of facilities. The goal is to produce cost savings. Clearly, vertical consolidation has the potential to change the nature of the market. The sheer size of these integrated networks makes them a potent force. An example of such a market is Minneapolis/St. Paul, in which three large health networks enroll over 75% of the managed care population. (Appendix A shows the evolution of managed care systems.)

But, Does It Save Money?

As the growth in managed care organizations continues, the key question remains unanswered: Does managed care contain costs? Theoretically, a larger number of health plans competing in the marketplace should result in lower costs and greater efficiency. Historically, however, this has not been the case in health care. No evidence indicates that increased competition has restrained the growth in health care spending. Part of the problem is that health care does not lend itself to market efficiency, which requires that price competition must reflect the true cost of resources. Health care products or services are highly individualized and personal; providers often do not compete effectively with one another on the basis of price, and most patients are insensitive to price because their insurance pays. Moreover, patients are not in a position to question what services their physician orders.

The concept of managed care is attractive, particularly among employers whose health care dollars are becoming a drain on corporate earnings. Fearful of doing nothing, most employers embrace the concept, even though the potential for cost containment is unclear. Employers, which are generally cautious about investing in new products, have adopted a lemming like approach to managed care.

Managed care's promise of holding down costs and improving care has wide appeal, but doubts have been expressed about its ability to do so. Cost-containment efforts occur primarily through controls on the use of expensive medical services and the reliance on network providers. HMOs traditionally have been successful in controlling hospital costs, eliminating unnecessary hospital admissions and decreasing length of stay; but, they have been less successful in reducing overall health costs. The cost reductions achieved by most managed care plans had been modest at best and highly variable. No plan has been able to slow the rate of inflation in costs, whatever their effect on the level of expenditures. Whatever was driving up the costs in the fee-for-service sector was driving them up in managed care as well. Also, by adding another layer of bureaucratic fat to the already corpulent system, these plans have created potentially more administrative costs and by their massive intrusive micromanagement have managed to increase the discontent of many patients and providers.

To date, a definitive evaluation of managed care does not exist because of the difficulty in obtaining comparable data and the constantly changing structure of managed care. Little evidence exists for the newer and typically less tightly controlled forms of managed care networks such as POS plans and EPOs. Few studies have been able to rigorously isolate savings resulting from managed care mechanisms from other factors that also influence costs. Patient selection and differences in benefit levels, for example, have been thought to account for differences in health plan costs. The healthier, younger individuals (who are less costly to care for) generally enroll in managed care plans, whereas those who consume large amounts of health resources are often reluctant to break established relationships with doctors to switch to a managed care plan. Selection bias does affect utilization and cost savings. Everything is relative and must be analyzed in context.

There is no doubt that managed care reduces the use of important diagnostic testing and the number of in-hospital days relative to the fee-for-service system. HMOs order fewer tests for patients with certain chronic diseases; yet, despite the lower testing rates, the quality of care in HMOs does not appear to suffer. Indeed, the most conspicuous distinction between HMOs and fee for service is the presence and absence, respectively, of normal economic market constraints on physicians' behavior. The fee-for-service system operated without the benefit of any inherent tendency toward efficiency. A Robert Wood Johnson/Harvard University School of Public Health study found that nonelderly sick individuals in managed care plans did have lower out-of-pocket expenses but more problems getting the health services or treatment that they, or their doctor, thought was necessary as compared to those in a fee-for-service plan. Patients in managed care plans also felt that they had more difficulty getting to see specialists than those in fee-for-service plans.

One approach to estimating savings from managed care is to compare the costs of a group enrolled in a managed care plan with a group of indemnity enrollees, careful to adjust for demographic factors and health status. Since such a study would take time and money, it is often more expedient (but less accurate) to rely on simple cost comparisons to support the claims of cost savings from managed care.

One study investigated HMO market penetration and hospital cost inflation in California. HMOs had been stimulating price competition in California hospital markets since 1983, which made this state an excellent laboratory for study. The California markets had been becoming increasingly more price competitive. The hypothesis was that health care markets with high levels of HMO penetration should exhibit lower costs than markets with low HMO penetration. The study found that HMOs can exert indirect effects on hospital behavior by stimulating more price competitive behavior on the part of other health insurance plans. *But,* the underlying dynamic of health care cost inflation, the development of new technologies and procedures, apparently had not been altered significantly.

To further illustrate how difficult it is to rein in health care costs, another study comparing hospital cost trends in Baltimore and the Twin Cities concluded that costs rose at virtually the same rate in Minnesota (10% annually) and Maryland (10.5% annually). Compared to the national average (11.2%), the regulatory strategy in Baltimore and the competitive strategy in Minneapolis/St. Paul had only a minor impact on controlling hospital expenditures.

To muddle the situation even more, it is instructive to cite a KPMG Peat Marwick study which evaluated financial and operational data on more than 3,600 hospitals. Findings revealed that markets with high levels of managed care experienced lower hospital costs, reduced lengths of stay and decreased mortality rates (after adjusting for the clinical condition of patients), while markets with less managed care showed minimal or no improvements in performance.

While the above may give employers something to be happy about, it should be explained that even if a managed care plan lowers utilization, the savings may not be passed on to the employer in lower premiums. *Shadow pricing,* which refers to the setting of premiums at a rate near the employers' other health plans regardless of actual cost, is known to exist. Surveys completed in the early 1990s found that managed care and indemnity premiums had experienced similar rates of growth, although HMO premium increases were marginally below indemnity plan premiums.

In summary, attempts to assess managed care plans have been hindered by the unavailability and incomparability of data on health plans. Some employers have reported that their managed care plans reduced costs. Others have found savings to be elusive. Most employers cannot confidently determine whether their managed care plans are resulting in savings. Employers are pressuring managed care entities to deliver the data so that key cost questions can be answered. They should demand no less!

What has managed care meant for physicians' incomes? A 1995 study found that for the first time, doctors' incomes are falling. The explanation is that managed care organizations have tightened their grip on reimbursement rates. Prices are falling in almost every market for both managed care premiums and compensation to physicians, indicating that managed care plans are succeeding in negotiating price discounts from providers.

What About Legal Issues?

The ascendancy of managed care has raised questions about concentration of power and antitrust issues. Although managed care has the potential to make health markets more efficient, there is the fear that oligopolies or monopolies could develop and prices and quality could be adversely affected. The complexities of the issue are beyond the scope of this book's purpose, but the questions raised are very serious and need to be addressed.

What about the exclusive nature of managed care? Physicians have become increasingly dependent on managed care contracts to maintain and sustain a flow of patients. Failure to be included in a managed care provider panel can severely affect the viability of a physician's practice. The issue of *any willing provider (AWP)* has generated heated debate. AWP laws provide that any physician willing to comply with the fee schedule and other requirements of a plan has a right to join that plan's provider panel. The managed care industry argues that the ability to select physicians is essential if quality and cost control are to be ensured. AWP laws would, in a sense, open up the network to all, thus defeating the purpose of a closed panel. There have been many court cases focusing on the tradeoffs between the rights of physicians to contract with plans and the necessity of plans to control the selection of their own provider panels.

Court cases regarding the issue of who is responsible for care have also been heard. (See Appendix B for a selected listing of cases.) Recent court rulings have found that utilization review or management firms can be held liable for injuries resulting from refusal to pay for further hospital care, and can be held accountable when medically inappropriate decisions result from defects in design or implementation of their cost-containment program or from malpractice committed by physicians retained by the HMO to furnish health care to enrollees. Such decisions increase managed care's exposure to physician malpractice suits. To what extent do managed care organizations avoid implementing or enforcing their internal standards, thus weakening their raison d'etre?

The growing area of managed care jurisprudence has found these organizations liable for their credentialing and contracting protocols and for defects in the design and implementation of cost-containment mechanisms that cause medically necessary services to be denied. Such defects could include sloppy program design, incompetent management, monitoring inadequate documentation, bad faith, or poor judgment of clinical or patient circumstances. These are serious questions which must be addressed.

Other legal challenges can be avoided by understanding ERISA's fiduciary requirements. HMO benefits that are part of a welfare plan come under ERISA's protection (self-insured plans are exempt). When an employer begins making benefit decisions, it becomes a fiduciary and therefore subject to certain provisions of ERISA. Employers can structure their health arrangements any way they want as long as self-dealing is not involved.

What Every Employer Should Ask

As managed care becomes more prevalent, and as controls are placed on utilization of services and patients' choice of providers, the employer must address how the changes in the marketplace will affect costs and quality of care. Some key questions that should be posed include:

- How do different types of managed care organizations control costs?
- How are the panel of providers selected and what are their credentials?
- What type of risk sharing do physicians undertake within the managed care organization?
- What effect do different types of risk sharing have on costs, access and quality?
- How does the managed care organization document client complaints?
- How much of the apparent cost savings from managed care has been passed on to the consumer?
- Have apparent cost savings represented a shift in costs, or a real reduction in the cost of medical care?
- How does the managed care organization monitor quality of care? Are providers held accountable for maintaining a standard of quality as part of a quality assurance program that meets the standards of the National Commission for Quality Assurance, for example?
- What is the degree of consumer choice? Is access to providers a problem?
- Is there an appeals process and, if so, how does it work?

Conclusion

The decrease in health care spending in 1994 and 1995 may be only a temporary lull, or it may represent the first sign of a restructuring spurred by managed care. It is much too early to draw conclusions given that cost studies have not isolated savings due to managed care mechanisms from savings due to other factors. Without proper adjustment for spending levels, savings due to other changes affecting the local health care market may be credited inappropriately to managed care. If not taken into account, confounding factors such as selection biases, benefit differences, and measurement of quality and cost factors, may create a distorted picture of the "success" of managed care.

One potential disadvantage of this system is the real possibility of a few organizations acquiring too much market power permitting them to maintain or raise prices and avoid lowering costs, thus negating the advantages of competitive markets. An imbalance of power could further squeeze providers, ignore the needs of the uninsured and poor, and create a monopolistic situation in which prices and quality could be adversely affected.

Employers must realize that accurate assessment of the effect of managed care requires data about costs as well as outcomes (including quality of care and satisfaction). To what extent does managed care contain costs by tightening regulatory controls and eligibility criteria for benefits? Deny recommended tests and hospital stays? Limit increases in fee schedules? There are so many unanswered questions, despite the unprecedented growth of managed care. One resource center, the Managed Care Information Center of Wall Township, New Jersey, was formed in 1994 in order to provide an authoritative, up-to-date resource center for monitoring the managed care market. But, the question of costs has become closely tied to the issue of quality and satisfaction (patient and provider). The following chapter will discuss this issue in greater detail.

APPENDIX A

How Markets Evolve

Editor's note: The following chart presents a view from APM Inc. and the University Hospital Consortium of stages of health care markets evolving as a result of reform and identifies markets in the various stages.

STAGE 1

Unstructured
—Little managed care
—Little hospital consolidation
—Few insurers active as providers
—Few physician groups
—Overuse of hospital care fuels oversupply of beds

Markets
—Nassau, Long Island, N.Y.
—Omaha, Neb.
—Syracuse, N.Y.
—Little Rock, Ark.
—Birmingham, Ala.
—Research Triangle, N.C.
—Newark, N.J.
—Shreveport, La.

STAGE 2

Loose framework
—Most managed care is discounted fee for service; by late Stage 2, some capitation
—Hospital consolidation begins
—Insurers begin to acquire partner or providers
—Physicians organize in groups; primary care doctors move toward large groups
—Oversupply of beds supports deep price discounts

Markets
—Louisville
—Miami
—Dallas/Ft. Worth
—Cincinnati
—Tampa/St. Petersburg
—Atlanta
—Orlando
—Cleveland
—St. Louis
—New York City
—New Orleans
—Indianapolis
—Nashville
—Philadelphia

STAGE 3

Consolidation
—Heavy managed care penetration, including government programs
—Managed care dominates payment scene
—Some capitation, especially of primary care M.D.s
—Hospital mergers accelerate
—Primary care doctors accelerate movement to groups; specialty doctors begin to form groups
—Plans begin dropping doctors, hospitals; shift in physician supply begins
—Managed care consolidation; providers, insurers begin to align
—Overcapacity begins to shrink
—Providers develop continuum of care

Markets
—Orange
—Milwaukee
—Portland
—San Francisco/Oakland
—Detroit
—Sacramento
—Denver
—Boston
—Salt Lake City
—Phoenix
—Seattle
—Washington, D.C.
—Houston
—Chicago

STAGE 4

Managed competition
—Employer coalitions buy health care
—Managed care payment dominates
—Little fee for service
—A few large health care players dominate
—Providers, insurers strongly align
—Doctors not in groups pushed out
—More pressure to eliminate beds
—Shift in physician supply
—Use of specialists and their fees driven down dramatically
—Networks develop full continuum of care, especially subacute
—Providers, insurers organize to serve covered lives
—More than 50% HMO penetration

Markets
—San Diego
—Minneapolis/St. Paul
—Los Angeles
—Worcester, MA

STAGE 5

Endgame
—Networks with market share form true partnerships with insurers
—Providers focus on their unique strengths
—Integrated systems manage patient populations

Markets
—No markets—yet

Source: Hospitals & Health Networks, March 5, 1995; APM Inc., and University Hospital Consortium, 1995.

APPENDIX B

Selected Legal Citings and Summaries Relevant
to Case Management and/or Managed Care

WICKLINE v. State of California, 228 Cal.Rptr.661 (Cal.Ct.App.1986)
Issue: Payer liability

After the state of California discounted her eligibility for MediCal payments following her physician's request for hospitalization extension, Lois Wickline suffered postoperative complications that necessitated the amputation of her leg. She sued the MediCal program (not the physician) and was awarded $500,000. This decision was reversed in 1989 with the court holding the physician ultimately responsible.

WILSON v. Blue Cross of Southern California and Blue Cross Blue Shield of Alabama and Western Medical Reserve, 271 Cal.Rptr. 876 (Cal.Ct.Appl.1990)
Issue: Authority to perform UR in CM, concurrence of physician and patient or family in treatment plan

Patient was admitted to a psychiatric hospital suffering from major depression, drug dependency and anorexia. He was discharged after third party payer funding was stopped. He subsequently committed suicide. Parents sued to recover on his behalf. The court of appeal held that: Contractor could be at least partially liable if negligent conduct was substantial factor in bringing about the suicide.

HUGHES v. Blue Cross of Northern California, 263 Cal.Rptr.850 (Cal.Ct.Appl.1989)
Issue: Bad faith

Following denial of coverage for a psychiatric hospitalization of the insured's son, a 1989 decision found that a UR decision was based on standards of medical necessity that were significantly more restrictive than community standards and that failure to properly investigate the insured's claim constituted bad faith.

LINTHICUM v. Nationwide Life Insurance Company, Ariz., 723 p.2d 675 (Ariz.1986)
Issue: Breach of contract and bad faith

Claims were reviewed four times by four different individuals and the procedure documented that review took into account the information submitted by the subscriber as well as additional information obtained by the insurer upon investigation of the claim. The court upheld retrospective denial of benefits.

BERGALIS v. CIGNA Dental Health Plan, Fla., 1991, no citation— settled out of court
Issue: Negligent referral, provider credentialing

Young college student visited dentist with AIDS and became HIV positive and died with no other exposure. Dentist was contracted provider. Case was settled out of court. Suit was against the HMO.

MOSHE v. Anchor Org. for Health Maintenance, 557 N.E.2nd 451 (Ill.App.Ct. 1990)
Issue: UR or CM activities may inhibit the ability of physicians to render care, questionable referral, questionable competence of agency

Patient's parents brought a medical malpractice action against a health services provider. The court dismissed all claims.

HARRELL v. Total Health Care, Inc., 781 S.W.2nd 58 (Mo.1989)
Issue: Negligent referral

In a 1989 Missouri appellate decision the court found that an IPA model could be held liable under the doctrine of corporate negligence for the alleged malpractice of a referral physician used by the plan on the basis that the plan had a duty to adequately check the credentials of its physicians.

NAZAY v. Miller, PA., 849 F.2nd 1323 (3d Cir. 1991)
Issue: Noncompliance with precert UR requirements of the plan

While the original ruling in this case supported a retiree who did not comply with precert UR requirements and was subsequently penalized for noncompliance by the plan, a subsequent ruling reversed that decision.

AETNA LIFE INSURANCE COMPANY v. Lavoie, Ala., 475 U.S. 813 (1986)
Issue: Bad faith

A 1986 Alabama decision in which a payer's decision to limit or deny payment for treatment which was made prior to complete review was found to constitute bad faith.

BOYD v. Albert Einstein Medical Center, 547 A.2d 1229 (Pa.Super.Ct. 1988)
Issue: Corporate negligence

In 1988, a Pennsylvania court found an independent practice association model HMO could be held vicariously liable for malpractice of an independently contracting physician.

SCHLEIER v. Kaiser Foundation Health Plan, 876 F.2d 174 (D.C.Cir. 1989)
Issue: Negligent referral

A 1989 District of Columbia court found the HMO liable for malpractice in the case of an outside consultant physician to whom a private care physician and a plan had referred a patient.

RULE v. Lutheran Hospital & Homes Soc'y of Am., 835 F.2d 1250 (8th Cir. 1987)
Issue: Provider liability for quality

In this action, the hospital was held liable for injuries to a baby caused by a physician during a breech birth. An administrator had incompletely checked basic credentials and the executive committee had merely rubber stamped the administrator's deficient investigation.

MORDECAI v. Blue Cross/Blue Shield of Alabama, 474 So.2d 95 (Ala.1985)
Issue: Breach of contract, bad faith

Where home health benefits were rejected, the subscriber sued for $4,596 seeking punitive damages for bad faith denial of claims and citing the insurer's failure in the UR process to consider portions of nurse notes to consult with treating nurses and physicians. The court upheld denial of claims.

ELSESSER v. Hospital of the Philadelphia College of Osteopathic Medicine, 802 F.Supp. 1286 (E.D. Pa. 1992)
Issue: Provider liability

The court held that the patient's negligence claims against an HMO seeking to hold it vicariously liable for actions of patient's primary physician, acting ostensibly as agent of HMO, were not preempted by ERISA.

CORCORAN v. United Healthcare, Inc., 91-3322 (U.S.Ct.App. 1992)

The court held that payment decisions may be medical decisions. Despite disclaimers, utilization management companies may be held liable for making medical decisions.

CHAPTER 5

Protecting Quality of Care

In a 1993 speech to Congress, President Clinton warned that "If we reform everything else in health care but fail to preserve and enhance the high quality of our medical care, we will have taken a step backward, not forward." As managed care continues to transform the health care system, and as the growth in health care costs appears to be abating, focus has shifted to the issue of quality. The importance of this noneconomic intangible cannot be minimized. While quality was not a prime reason for the creation of managed care networks, its quantification is of paramount importance to their survival. The purchasers of care (the consumers) are rightfully demanding documentation from managed care providers of both the economic and noneconomic factors associated with the delivery of care. In fact, the intense competition in the field is a major driving force behind the rush to identify, gather and analyze data.

In order to measure and assess performance measures such as quality of care, outcomes and patient satisfaction, the system is gradually transforming itself into an information-based and information-driven system. Information has become a critical factor in health care marketing and is a necessary component for consumer decision making. To what extent does managed care deliver high-quality health care? To what extent does managed care affect physicians' ability to provide high-quality patient care? To what extent do some managed care organizations perform better than others in terms of better quality and reduced costs? The answers to such questions, unfortunately, are not readily apparent; but, they are questions that each purchaser of care should ask when trying to decide which managed care product to offer to employees. The key is to find the correct balance between cost containment and quality of care. Do not be swayed by the low bid of some managed care companies or by anecdotal examples of good care. Demand data, proof, of their assertions.

This chapter will discuss the issues surrounding quality management and managed care's ability and commitment to ensuring quality. It will focus on means of assessing quality, patient satisfaction and clinical outcomes.

Quality

Defining *quality of care* requires a definition of the attributes of the care provided as well as a criteria for what constitutes good care. We all know bad care when we experience it; but, what about the less obvious indicators of less-than-optimal care? Defining the term, much less measuring it, is not so easy. *Quality* is such a nebulous concept that forming a consensus on how to measure it has challenged many researchers over the past years. What constitutes quality and how utilization and costs are affected are interrelated issues as yet unresolved by research or policy. For purposes herein, *quality* will refer to the degree to which health care services meet the patients' needs, expectations and standards of care. It is important to realize that quality is not defined for a single patient; rather, measurements rely on all of the providers' patients.

Most of the early studies relied on Donabedian's approach to assessing quality and, to a certain extent, his method is still the gold standard. Donabedian described three approaches to the assessment of quality: observation of structure, process and outcome. *Structure* refers to the basic characteristics of the health care delivery system such as the credentials of the staff, board certification, affiliation with a medical school, the availability of specialized services, the condition of the facilities and the equipment. *Process* describes what the providers do as they take care of their patients. *Measures* include appropriate prescription of drugs, appropriate selection of patients for surgery, documentation of history and physical exams, and the like. Assessment of process, that is, how care is delivered, is more intangible but very important. Some examples of recently developed measures of process, which will be discussed subsequently, include utilization review, practice guidelines, total quality management and disease management. Process is usually related to outcome. *Outcome,* which has assumed heightened interest, refers to what happens to the patient as a result of the medical care received. The most commonly used outcome measures include morbidity, mortality and patient satisfaction. Did the patient get better? Did the patient die? Did the patient develop complications? In short, what happened to the patient after receiving treatment? Measures include recovery time from surgery, complications/infections, death, and the like. Of course, researchers account for severity of illness when assessing outcome.

How do managed care organizations rank in terms of quality of care? Again, the field is rapidly amassing data to answer this question and, to a large extent, the jury is still out. Recent studies, however, have shown that HMO and indemnity plans provided enrollees with roughly comparable quality of care, according to process and outcome measures. The studies' findings were clear that the quality of care of moderately ill patients with common diseases was not adversely affected in an HMO setting. The researchers independently found no evidence that any one system of care or physician specialty achieved consistently better two-year or four-year outcomes.

Means of Ensuring Quality

One of the greatest challenges of managed care is to ensure quality of care. Because purchasers choose plans on the basis of quality, cost and excellence, such variables must be documented; i.e., value for dollars expended must be quantified. Managed care organizations must be able to show that quality will be safeguarded and that fears of undertreatment and discrimination against consumers with costly medical problems are unfounded. Any system that attempts to cut costs without safeguarding quality most certainly will find itself embroiled in litigation.

Utilization Review

During the 1980s, a large bureaucracy of *utilization review (UR)* firms was spawned. Their focus was to assess the appropriateness and/or necessity of care in order to monitor quality and help contain costs. For the most part, these UR firms were established on behalf of health benefits purchasers to manage costs through a case-by-case assessment of the clinical justification for proposed care. The most prevalent UR activities included preadmission or precertification, concurrent review, discharge planning, second surgical opinions, disability case management, psychiatric review and case management.

The use of a pre-established review criteria to make recommendations regarding care served as the core function of UR firms. Most UR firms rely on a nurse to provide UR services, although in some cases physicians are also involved in the decision. Review criteria are based on clinical indicators that relate to either a specific diagnosis, the intensity of care required or a combination of the two. That is, criteria would be developed for reviewing a patient being admitted to a hospital for diabetes (a diagnosis), a patient experiencing chest pain (a symptom) or a patient requiring a surgical procedure. In each case, the criteria would indicate which medical services are appropriate. Just about every UR firm has a quality assurance monitoring process to ensure that their staff make appropriate decisions.

There are times when the physician's proposed care would not conform to the UR criteria. The case would then be referred to another reviewer for a second level review and a recommendation would be made. Failure to comply with UR recommendations would result in a penalty; therefore, physicians had to be sure that the proposed care would be approved by the UR firm. The nature of this system increased the likelihood that an appeal/challenge would be made. The previous chapter discussed the legal exposure and listed some key cases. Plan penalties that have been designed on the basis of actual data, even if the data is not the plan's own, are less likely to be called into question than those designed more intuitively. Nevertheless, the UR firms must be aware that they would be liable if the court ruled against them.

Utilization Management

Just as health care policy is constantly evolving, UR firms, too, are restructuring their focus. Rather than performing reviews, most are now engaged in *utilization management (UM)*. Whereas the primary focus of UR is to contain costs, UM looks at cost, quality and outcome—the focus is on medical effectiveness (quality/outcome) and efficiency (cost). The objective is to move from identifying outliers to improving average levels of performance. Crucial to UM is the application of clinically valid criteria, policies and guidelines in order to quantify outcomes and conduct data analyses. The development of a database which combines UM and claims data is required to assess quality and cost savings.

By the mid-1990s, virtually every managed care organization offers some UM services. Scores of independent companies provide UM services and therein lies a problem. Neither administrative processes nor clinical criteria for review are highly standardized. In fact, there are differences in assessing the appropriateness of specific services, in qualification of the staff, in training and supervision, in the ability to analyze data, and in the appeals process. It soon became obvious that there had to be some order, some standard put in place.

Report Cards and Benchmarking

Most cost-conscious purchasers believe it is critical to hold UM organizations accountable for their performance, but there is still a lot of variability in how plans measure performance. Report cards have been touted as a means of highlighting one's performance and helping the purchaser of care to select an organization that would be the best buy for their benefit dollar, but there are problems inherent in this system. So far, it is the providers who are doing their own grading: United Healthcare, U.S. Healthcare and several other HMOs have published their respective report cards. This is all well and good, but there are variations in design and analysis, which complicate things. A standardized report card is needed in order to make proper sense out of all of the data. Beware of players blowing their own horns!

Concerns about the quality of the UR and UM organizations prompted the industry to establish a voluntary accreditation program. In 1990 the Utilization Review Accreditation Commission was established to develop quality assurance standards and to accredit organizations that sought this distinction. This commission was created by the American Medical Association, the American Hospital Association and others to provide a means of assessing and evaluating the scores of firms in business.

National standards for prospective and concurrent hospital reviews were published in 1990 and included such requirements as having only licensed or certified and trained staff conduct utilization reviews; preparing, with physician involvement, written clinical criteria/protocols for determining the appropriateness of care; having clinical review criteria for determining the appropriateness of care periodically updated; and having an appeals process.

The National Committee for Quality Assurance (NCQA), an independent review organization, was formed to foster the development of internal systems for quality assurance. It is an accreditation program and publishes reviewer guidelines. The NCQA Users' Group, comprised of purchasers, consumers and union representatives, reviews existing standards and makes recommendations about new ones. NCQA, in collaboration with health plan representatives and employers, has taken the lead in designing performance assessment by developing and marketing the Health Plan Employer Data and Information Set (HEDIS 2.0).

HEDIS 2.0, a standardized performance measure, is used to document value and identify areas that need improvement by systematizing the process of care. Implicit in HEDIS 2.0 is the application of standardized definitions and specific methodologies to derive measures of performance, including quality, access to care, patient satisfaction, changes in membership, utilization, finance and management activities (i.e., provider credentialing and utilization review). This instrument permits a user to examine trends within its own plan as well as compare its results to others to see how it ranks (benchmarking). HEDIS 2.0 has been accepted by many state health agencies and numerous corporations. At this writing, a new HEDIS 3.0 is being finalized. This version will include outcomes measures, which are supposed to be more patient oriented and stress more multifaceted data gathering.

Other instruments are being developed in this data-driven environment. A new group of purchasers and consumers is developing a set of patient-oriented quality measures that are intended to assess health plan performance in a two-tier system of accountability. Measurement of how well the health system provides services to its entire patient population will be complemented by measurement of how effectively the system provides care for people when they are ill. The group, the Foundation for Accountability, hopes to have its measures released in 1996.

Even though the industry has set up accrediting entities to police itself, employers, the purchasers of care, must demand an accounting from UR and UM firms to decide for themselves whether the program is achieving its objectives. Taking matters into their own hands, several leading corporations have formed a national coalition (National HMO Purchasing Coalition) to identify and select high-quality, cost-efficient HMOs. In order to evaluate the quality-of-care issue, the coalition conducts site visits and relies on member satisfaction surveys.

Outcomes Research

Outcomes research, another key concept of the 1990s, is a very broad term. It essentially seeks to understand the link between outcomes and medical care to better distinguish which patients will benefit from specific types of care, which treatments to reimburse. Outcomes include the traditional measures of mortality and morbidity, assessment of physical function, mental well-being and aspects of health-related quality of life. Outcomes research also includes the collection of data that can be used to compare the quality of care delivered by physicians and managed care organizations. That is, monitoring the quality of providers over time, identifying high-quality providers, identifying providers who deliver the highest quality of care at the lowest cost. But, there are dangers in placing too much trust in the results. Data upon which the results are based may not be reliable, generalizable or systematically collected. Comparisons must be based on credible case mix adjustments of outcomes data, for example.

The goals of outcomes management are both to improve cost-effectiveness and maintain quality of care. Yes, these are noble and sensible goals, but until we reach the point where we have standardization or uniformity of measures to gauge quality to determine what optimal guidelines are, it will be difficult to make sense out of the findings. First, *outcomes* needs to be defined. Are we looking at mortality? Length of stay? Complications? Restoration of functional status? Long term? Short term?

Essentially, outcomes should pertain to some treatment intervention (the outcome should be the product or be causally linked with the treatment intervention) and be associated with advancing the patient's well-being.

Outcomes research has been hailed as one of the best means of solving the problems of quality and cost. It permits the monitoring of the quality of providers, identifying providers who deliver the highest quality of care at the lowest cost as well as targeting low-quality providers in an effort to improve quality. With such results, the consumer will know more about the care they are buying. In a sense, outcomes research represents a sensible approach to the assessment of medical care. What is needed, however, is an evaluation of whether the efforts ultimately achieve their goals of improving quality and reducing costs.

Practice Guidelines

Numerous studies have uniformly found that many health care services delivered in the United States are inappropriate or ineffective and that the use of procedures across different regions, even within small areas of a region, vary without any apparent medical justification. Indeed, the literature clearly shows that individuals with the same basic condition often receive different evaluations or treatments. Such variations are potentially costly and may lead to different outcomes.

Because hospital stays and unnecessary or inappropriate practice are so expensive, the use of practice guidelines (also called clinical pathways) has intensified in an effort to contain costs and promote quality care. Practice guidelines are systematically developed statements, based on the best available scientific evidence and expert opinion, designed to assist practitioners about appropriate health care for specific clinical circumstances; i.e., to assist clinicians and patients in making decisions about health care, thereby enhancing quality and effectiveness and achieving improved outcomes for patients. Most measurements derived from clinical practice guidelines are process measurements. That is, the assessment of process measures can provide information about the sustainability of that performance and about the relationship of the process to the outcome.

The system requires physicians to base their treatment plan on information from statistical analyses of large databases. The focus is to determine the most efficient and effective treatment plan. But, some physicians feel that practice guidelines bring the profession a step closer to cookbook medicine. Is it too rigid a system? Patients, after all, present with individual and complex medical circumstances; however, what practice guidelines attempt to do is set practice parameters to reduce inappropriate and costly care, which we all know exists. Practice guidelines are not intended to promote a rigid adherence to a specific "right" way of providing care. Rather, they serve as a means of evaluating overall quality of care.

Guidelines are developed usually by a panel of physician experts in their field to facilitate clinical decision making. Milliman and Robertson, a Seattle-based actuarial and consulting firm, is one of the most influential among the numerous firms who write standards for specific procedures. Their guidelines, based on findings from published studies in academic journals as well as from medical chart reviews, are designed to address when and for how long the patient should be hospitalized, in what type of facility, and what the usual and expected costs of care should be. The objective is to find the most effective and efficient means of treating patients; the guidelines should be used as recommendations for treating patients without complications. Opponents of the concept complain that guidelines are tantamount to practicing cookbook medicine. Others feel that UR and UM firms take the guidelines and apply them as a gold standard without taking into account that medicine is an inexact science and patients differ.

The micromanagement of care can be very frustrating in certain situations. For example, 1995 witnessed a minirevolt among obstetrical patients and their obstetricians. Many managed care organizations required that the new mother and her newborn leave the hospital one day after delivery. It was only after data were collected to show that mother and baby often did not do well after being discharged so soon after delivery that managed care organizations relented and allowed the extra day. In this instance, the doctors and their patients showed that the managed care rules were sacrificing the patients' best interests and in some cases costing more money as a result of readmissions.

Since practice guidelines address appropriate treatment of a condition or disease and since each individual patient is different, there logically are many diverging pathways or sequences of care that have to be allowed for. Each pathway would have a more specific guideline recommendation for a more narrowly defined and homogeneous group of patients. There theoretically would be numerous pathways for a patient presenting with chest pain, each refining clinical and demographic characteristics, which would take into account risk factors and severity of illness. Clearly, there must be some clinical flexibility; for some patients, clinicians may justifiably decide that clinical practice guidelines do not apply.

The U.S. Chamber of Commerce supports the use of medical guidelines in an effort to produce a health care system in which medical care would be more consistently effective and largely devoid of unnecessary and needlessly expensive treatment. Despite the popularity of relying on guidelines, the jury is still out as to whether better and more cost-effective care can be delivered. Indeed, it is important to find answers to some very basic questions before we can say that a managed care organization is providing the best care: How do deviations from a treatment recommendation affect patient outcome? How do variations in practice style, use of tests and procedures, and discussion of treatment options affect patient outcome and patient satisfaction? How cost-effective is the use of guidelines in outcomes research?

Total Quality Management (TQM)

Total quality management (TQM) is derived from the principles of continuous improvement. The focus on quality management has become a continuous process in contrast to the more traditional approach to management problem solving. The emphasis is on improving the overall level of performance and achieving greater consistency. This approach emphasizes the need for teamwork in identifying patient needs, meeting patient needs and evaluating the success of care. TQM is designed to "do the right thing" and "do it right." It addresses every dimension of the provision of a service and the relative contributions of each to quality outcomes. Communication, education, quality control methods and employee involvement are critical components of TQM. Implementing TQM is more difficult than other quality assurance mechanisms; as such, not all organizations would benefit from this approach to quality measurement. The advantages and disadvantages as well as barriers to implementation should be carefully weighed.

Disease Management

Judging by the increasing number of seminars and publications on *disease management (DM),* it appears that this new concept is growing in popularity. DM is based on a comprehensive look at the entire pattern of care for a particular disease and the result of that care. It acknowledges that each disease has its own natural course, its own set of cost drivers, and that the individual components of care (and concomitant costs) are interrelated. DM is a data-driven concept based in outcomes research.

Theoretically, DM focuses on cost components within each disease such as providers of care, drugs and ancillary tests. The goal is to affect the outcome of the disease and the long-term cost. Partnerships are often required to manage the treatment plan. Disease management also helps individuals assess their personal risk for disease and offers tools to avoid those diseases; at-risk individuals can be offered educational and clinical support to help change behavior and to avoid high utilization of the costlier health care services. Practice guidelines are relied upon but a multidisciplinary team of providers refine and simplify the guidelines to manage the patient. Overutilization of services is discouraged and patient involvement encouraged.

The goals, then, of DM are not particularly revolutionary; i.e., to reduce medical expenditures by:
- Facilitating diagnosis
- Maximizing clinical effectiveness
- Eliminating unnecessary or ineffective care
- Using most cost-efficient diagnostics and therapeutics
- Maximizing efficiency of care delivery
- Continually improving care.

DM usually is found in sophisticated managed care markets as opposed to markets in which managed care is not yet strong. Generally, the program revolves around a drug product(s) in conjunction with treatment for a chronic disease such as asthma, diabetes, hypertension and depression. Patients with chronic diseases account for a disproportionate amount of health plan costs. With better management of the condition and with patient education, it is hypothesized that more effective care could be rendered at reduced costs.

Early efforts of DM have focused on *pharmacy benefits managers (PBMs)* as resource individuals who use their databases to model drug expenditure patterns and target high-risk or high utilizing patients for intervention/education. The growing integration of medical claims data and pharmacy claims data increases the potential effect of PBMs. Examples of PBMs are Medco, Diversified and PCS. In fact, pharmaceutical manufacturers are devoting substantial resources to DM; for them, DM is a good opportunity to demonstrate the value of pharmacy as an integrated element of treatment.

Does DM save money? To date, there is little evidence to show that DM saves money. However, it takes a long time to implement a DM program The rationale is that since most chronic diseases are expensive to treat and typically involve large practice variation, in the long run costs could be reduced by better management. Such thinking is hard to refute. Maybe DM will lead to a better health care system; time will tell.

Summary

Ironically, the field of quality assurance has moved from one characterized by a dearth of data to one in which there are now scores of performance measures, report cards, quality indicators and patient satisfaction surveys, each designed to assess quality. Indeed, groups looking to assess quality need not reinvent the wheel. There are scores of surveys and research instruments available to consider. (See the appendix.) However, it is imperative that the findings be interpreted with a jaundiced eye. You should understand how the survey was conducted, on whom and for what purpose. A major problem is that there is disagreement over the type of questions to ask, how to frame them and how to present the results. Often, questions are phrased in a leading way and results are interpreted in the most favorable light. That is, reports and surveys can be misleading and subjective. The field is still in its infancy and the buyer should beware. *Be sure you know what you are buying.*

Patient Satisfaction

The patient, the consumer of care, plays an important role in assessing quality. By expressing preferences and by offering feedback, the patient helps define the meaning of quality in a technical sense; through expression of satisfaction or dissatisfaction, the patient/consumer passes a judgment about many aspects of the structure, process and outcome of care. In particular, patients' satisfaction with their medical care is considered a central factor in understanding the functioning of a health care system and in assessing the quality of care rendered. Insofar as that satisfaction is based on a patient's assessment of the care received, satisfaction is potentially a direct and powerful indicator of system performance.

Managed care organizations, which must compete on cost and quality, realize that consumers are more sophisticated about the type of care they receive, are generally more knowledgeable and prefer to be involved in the care experience. The literature is clear that satisfied patients are more likely to remain with their provider, keep appointments, comply with treatment protocol, refer others to their doctor and use services. Taken as a whole, these characteristics should result in better medical care and improved outcomes.

Most studies on patient satisfaction report that the majority say that they are satisfied with their medical care, whatever form of delivery. A 1995 study conducted by the Group Health Association of America found that HMO and fee-for-service patients report similar satisfaction levels with their care, regardless of their self-reported health status and age group. Often, however, it is impossible to tell exactly what is being measured. Different or undefined concepts of patient satisfaction, and different study procedures, make it difficult to generalize results meaningfully. Further, when a patient says that the service is satisfactory, does it mean that he or she is satisfied? If the patient says that he or she is satisfied, does it mean that the care is good? For example, a patient may be quite happy with his or her congenial doctor who is providing inappropriate care!

Expressions of satisfaction, or dissatisfaction, may be reflecting a level of expectation, and expectations may differ according to varying socio-demographic and socioeconomic characteristics. Moreover, an individual may be satisfied in general terms, but have a number of specific dissatisfactions. Dissatisfactions with costs, professional competence, communication with the providers, or location, for example, are factors in a patient's decision to change providers. As such, any consideration of satisfaction must include consideration of dissatisfaction as well, and take into account patient characteristics.

Factors shown to be related to patient satisfaction include socio-demographic characteristics (age, social class, ethnicity), health status, and attitudes and expectations concerning medical care. Studies show that those patients with low expectations were less satisfied with the services they received, and that patients tend to be more satisfied with their care if their providers' behavior conformed to expectations. There is no consensus about which of these factors is most important.

The way in which care is organized and financed has been shown to be related to patient satisfaction. This point is particularly important to managed care organizations. Accessibility, availability and convenience of care are highly correlated with patient satisfaction. Having a regular source of care and relationship with the same provider is positively related to satisfaction with care. Regarding the technical aspects of care, overall the research implies that satisfaction is related to perceptions of technical skills and qualifications, but perceived interpersonal and communication skills (doctor-patient interaction) account for more of the variation in patient satisfaction. Patients tend to be more satisfied if they perceive that their doctor is caring and sensitive to their needs.

Patient satisfaction can be used to monitor the quality of care as well as to market/promote the organization. The two are not mutually exclusive. The best marketing tactics will not succeed in the long term if patients do not find the quality of care to be as advertised. Patient satisfaction and quality-of-care issues should dictate marketing strategies, not the other way around.

In summary, reliance on patient satisfaction surveys offers an excellent means for patients to comment on the care they receive and for the provider to assess how it can improve its services. It is important to periodically survey individuals to obtain a more objective view. That is, those who are unhappy or dissatisfied will generally make their feelings known, usually loud and clear, while those who are happy or pleased tend not to express themselves as vociferously or as frequently.

Conclusion

The science of measuring quality has advanced tremendously over the past decade, and its importance has grown immensely in the competitive managed care environment. Correlating costs and quality to outcomes has assured heightened interest as well as spawned a new field for researchers. Applying outcomes assessment in markets is big business! Too many managed care organizations had stressed only cost incentives, but now realize that data on outcomes are the key factor consumers are seeking. The market is rapidly becoming data driven, and managed care organizations prosper or die on their documented ability to contain costs without sacrificing quality of care.

What, then, is the consumer supposed to do? How should the mounds of data (both useful and otherwise) be interpreted? While the basic coverage is often similar, it is helpful to look for the little extras that can make a difference (home care services, coverage of preexisting conditions, and the like). After reading the promotional material and plan contract, visit the clinics and offices. Check state records to see what proportion of people disenroll from a plan. Find out what fraction of patient complaints have been upheld by state insurance departments. Find out how many primary doctors and specialists are affiliated with the plan. Be sure you understand what sort of approval a plan requires before a primary care doctor can refer a patient to a specialist. Find out the procedure for appealing a plan's denial of treatment that a patient believes is necessary. Understand those treatments deemed by the plan as "experimental" and therefore not covered. Most importantly, is the plan stable enough that it is likely to pay claims quickly and keep their doctors happy?

The purchasers of care must become more sophisticated in order to intelligently make important decisions regarding the type of health care package which is right for their organization. Industry report cards, performance measures, and the like will become increasingly important as a means of consumer selection of managed care providers.

APPENDIX

Guide to Medical Quality Measurement Systems

NATIONAL COMMITTEE FOR QUALITY ASSURANCE (NCQA)
2000 L Street NW, Suite 500
Washington, DC 20036
202-955-3500
> HEDIS 2.0 measurement, which is a standardized set of performance measures. It is used by many corporations.

GROUP HEALTH ASSOCIATION OF AMERICA (GHAA)
1129 20th Street NW, Suite 600
Washington, DC 20036
202-778-3249
> Developed a consumer satisfaction instrument.

THE HMO GROUP
100 Albany Street, Suite 130
New Brunswick, NJ 08901
908-220-1388
> Developed a measurement tool to compare performance among health plans and to identify areas for improvement.

CLEVELAND HEALTH QUALITY CHOICE PROGRAM
1137 Euclid Avenue, Suite 741
Cleveland, OH 44115
> Developed a patient viewpoint survey and a risk-adjusted patient satisfaction survey.

EMPLOYEE HEALTH CARE VALUE SURVEY
Coopers and Lybrand
One International Place
Boston, MA 02110
Contact: Harris M. Allen Jr.
> Developed a consumer-based measurement index to assess performance and quality, accessibility, satisfaction, functional status and well-being.

IOWA HEALTH SURVEY
Health Policy Corp. of Iowa
2 Ruan Center, Suite 300
Des Moines, IA 50309-3774
515-244-1211
> Survey to assess quality.

PACIFIC BUSINESS GROUP ON HEALTH
33 New Montgomery Street, Suite 1450
San Francisco, CA 94105
415-281-8660
> Health Plan Value Check survey measures health status, use of preventive services and satisfaction.

MARYLAND QUALITY INDICATOR PROJECT
Maryland Hospital Association
1301 York Road, Suite 800
Luterville, MD 21093-6087
410-321-6200
> Established indicators that would allow hospitals to compare quality of services with other hospitals; indicators could force hospitals to consider all factors surrounding individual and comparative performances in specific areas, and then determine whether their methods are appropriate.

AMERICAN COLLEGE OF PHYSICIANS' CLINICAL EFFICACY ASSESSMENT PROJECT
American College of Physicians
6th Street at Race
Philadelphia, PA 19106-1572
215-351-2840
> Goal is to determine clinical efficacy of medical procedures, drugs, devices and other technologies in order to assist physicians and patients in decision making, effectiveness, and costs of existing and new technologies and practices.

PRACTICE PARAMETERS PARTNERSHIP AND FORUM
American Medical Association
515 N. State Street
Chicago, IL 60610
312-464-5928
> Goal is to coordinate activities of the medical profession in the development, dissemination and implementation of practice parameters.

In addition to the above mentioned, there are other numerous outcomes studies underway. An excellent source is the *Medical Outcomes and Guidelines Sourcebook.*

CHAPTER 6

Wellness and Health Promotion

It is hard to deny that most of us would be healthier if we took better care of ourselves. While intellectually all of us know what we should do to live a healthier life, we also know that health habits are extremely difficult to change. After all, if it were easy, the number of cigarette smokers, for example, would be greatly diminished; the number of overweight individuals would be nil. There is considerable evidence showing that most lifestyle behaviors can be modified. One can increase one's physical activity, take up measures to control blood pressure and cholesterol levels, reduce alcohol intake and reduce stress. For other factors, however, it is not so easy. Biology and genetics play a significant role in the management of body weight, for example.

Because diseases and conditions related to unhealthy lifestyles account for a large portion of medical bills, one of the means of managing costs (and improving the health and well-being of employees at the same time) entails promoting a healthier personal lifestyle. The objectives of health promotion and wellness programs are to help individuals change their lifestyle to achieve a state of optimal health and well-being. Lifestyle changes can be facilitated through a

91

combination of efforts to enhance awareness, change behavior and create environments that support good health practices.

Health status and the way the body reacts to diseases are shaped by life experiences and health habits. Years of poor health habits are a tremendous drain on the health care system and contribute to employee absenteeism, failure to work at full potential and lost productivity. It is striking that almost all of the risk factors identified with the major causes of sickness and death are behavioral or have a large behavioral component on which technology-intensive medical care has limited impact.

There is no doubt that medical advances and changing lifestyles have helped improve the health, vitality and well-being of many, regardless of age. New technology and medical breakthroughs have helped contribute to increased life expectancy; however, with this gain in additional years, many are living with some form of chronic disability such as heart problems, high blood pressure, cancers and respiratory conditions. Many of these chronic diseases could have been prevented had the individual maintained good health habits early in life.

The Centers for Disease Control and Prevention estimates that over half of all premature deaths in adults in the United States are from lifestyle-related causes. Logically, in order to prevent these premature deaths, we need to address the causes, which include smoking, poor eating habits, sedentary lifestyles and poor management of stress. Looking at the leading causes of deaths in the United States affirms the fact that lifestyle priorities are the most important contributing factors to the majority of leading causes of death (see Table I). Approximately one-quarter of premature deaths are a result of human biology and/or genetic defects while one-fifth are a result of environmental factors. Less than one-fifth of premature deaths are from problems that are treatable through traditional medical care.

This chapter presents an overview of the health status of Americans and how wellness/health promotion programs can be integrated into an organization's benefits program. Discussion will explore the importance of health promotion as well as the costs and benefits of wellness programs. Specifically, are health promotion/wellness programs worth the investment? What type of programs work best? Will such programs be utilized by the employees?

Measures of Health

Historically, the health of a population has been assessed by means of mortality rates. The assumption is that any reduction in mortality reflects a reduction in morbidity (improved health). Mortality rates, however, shed

TABLE I

Leading Causes of U.S. Deaths, 1992

	% of Total Deaths
Heart Disease*	33.1
Cancers*	23.9
Stroke*	6.6
Chronic Obstructive Pulmonary Diseases*	4.2
Accidents*	4.2
Pneumonia and Influenza	3.5
Diabetes	2.3
HIV Infection/AIDS*	1.5
Suicide	1.4
Homicide	1.2

* Denotes that lifestyle is the leading cause of death for these diseases.
Source: Centers for Disease Control and Prevention/National Center for Health Statistics.

little light on the incidence and prevalence of illness or the impact of illness on functioning. Today, studies of health status focus not only on mortality rates, but also on the prevalence of chronic and acute diseases, impairments, short- and long-term disability, and self-perception of health.

Trends in Mortality

Since the turn of the century, trends in mortality reflect both advances in medicine and public health measures. The introduction of sulfamide drugs and antibiotics as well as improvements in sanitation and hygiene, as well as the development of immunizations, helped eliminate high mortality from acute infections, parasitic diseases and the like. Rather than dying from pneumonia, tuberculosis, influenza and infections, we now die from heart diseases, cancers and stroke. Death from these conditions reflects years of abuse from smoking, stressful lifestyles, diet and environmental factors. Even though modern methods of early detection and more efficient treatment modalities have helped individuals survive longer, for the most part, these conditions are chronic—rarely is one cured.

Trends in Morbidity

Whereas the statistics clearly show that we are living longer, are we actually healthy? The "killer diseases" are controlled by modern medicine, but the treatment results in substantial costs over an individual's remaining years. Other chronic diseases such as respiratory conditions (bronchitis, emphysema and sinusitis) and chronic digestive conditions (lower bowel problems, gallbladder problems) account for more than 80% of all disability and an estimated 80% of all health care expenditures, excluding the more intangible costs of pain, suffering, lost productivity and absenteeism.

For the most part, we can do something to prevent many conditions from developing. Although Americans, in general, eat less fat now than in the past, we still eat too much of those foods high in saturated fats. The same is true for foods high in sugars, cholesterol, salt and sodium. Conversely, we tend to eat less of those foods that are beneficial—those high in fiber, for example.

We tend not to exercise regularly, we tend not to control our stress and we tend not to give up habits which we know are unhealthy.

Costs of Unhealthy Behaviors

Every study investigating health risks and their impact on medical costs concludes that significant differences exist in the cost of medical care by health risk status. Table II shows that a person with an elevated level of risk generally uses more medical care than an individual with a low-risk status. Those who smoke, for example, experience one-third higher claims costs than nonsmokers. Those who are overweight have 143% higher hospital inpatient utilization than those in a healthy weight range. Those with poor eating habits generate 41% higher claims costs than those with good eating habits. While these statistics are from claims experience for employees of the Chrysler Corp., they probably reflect similar findings from any company in the United States. Another survey also concluded that significant differences exist in the utilization and costs of medical care by health risk status, with high-risk individuals utilizing more medical care and generating higher claims costs than others of lower risk. Those who do not wear seat belts regularly experience 54% more hospital days than those who do wear seat belts. Those who are hypertensive are 68% more likely to have claims in excess of $5,000 per year than those who are not hypertensive.

Simple Steps Can Be Taken

Simply educating individuals about the risks of their behavior and/or lifestyle, asking people to change these habits, is not the most effective means of modifying behavior. Compounding the problem is the fact that Americans tend to favor programs that will reap immediate rewards or improvement. People say that they want to change behavior to improve their

TABLE II

Total Average Monthly Claim per Participant and Annual Utilization

Health Characteristic	Total Costs[1]		Hospital Inpatient[2]		Hospital Outpatient[3]	
	Elevated Risk	Low Risk	Elevated Risk	Low Risk	Elevated Risk	Low Risk
Smoking	$121.94	$93.44	288	190	1,012	949
Weight control	125.05	90.83	420	173	1,087	914
Exercise	104.34	96.32	223	209	1,039	925
Alcohol use	93.08	103.66	221	185	952	970
Driving habits	103.26	94.43	213	201	1,015	930
Eating habits	111.12	79.26	236	174	1,033	846
Stress	112.44	89.52	218	193	1,178	871
Mental health	101.02	89.19	200	193	984	916
Cholesterol	96.13	96.29	211	195	914	988
Blood pressure	103.46	95.02	248	200	925	968

Source: Brink, Milliman & Robinson Inc. and StayWell Health Management Systems Inc., 1995.

1. Includes hospital inpatient, outpatient, physician, radiology/pathology and other costs.
2. Days per 1,000.
3. Services per 1,000.

lives right now, not some time in the future. The focus tends to be on quality of life, not on longevity per se. Americans also tend to be confused by the conflicting results of studies investigating the relationships between different health behaviors. Medical information from studies reported in the news media can be contradictory, resulting in frustration and bewilderment. Should one eat butter or margarine? Will moderate exercise suffice, or does only rigorous exercise make a difference? Do vitamin supplements make a difference or not? While the complexity of intervention studies leads to confusion, the literature is quite clear that there are simple steps that can be taken, which would have an immediate and profound effect on health status and on medical costs.

- Do not smoke cigarettes.
- Do not abuse drugs.
- Drink alcohol moderately or do not drink at all.
- Exercise three or more times a week.
- Maintain recommended weight range.
- Eat sensibly—avoid eating too much salt, sodium or high-cholesterol foods, and try to eat more fiber.
- Take steps to control or reduce stress.
- Check your blood pressure at least once a year.

- Women should have a Pap smear taken every one to two years and examine their breasts at least once a month for signs of cancer.
- Wear seat belts all the time when you drive.

While these recommendations certainly have been suggested by others, and while intellectually most of us know that we should be following this advice, "easier said than done" best summarizes the sentiment. And, that is why health promotion programs are so important. It is much easier to comply with these recommendations if there is a collective, group effort. If one is motivated to stick with the plan, if one is encouraged along the way, the likelihood of achieving one's goal is greater.

Objectives of Health Promotion

The goals of health promotion are to reduce premature mortality and to improve health status. Educational programs, counseling, effecting an increase in awareness of relationships between specific health behaviors and disease, and encouraging appropriate health behavior modifications are all mechanisms to promote healthy behaviors. The concept entails promoting measures that are designed to encourage behavioral and environmental changes, eliminate risk hazards, and raise individual fitness and good health. Since few have the strength to diligently live the "healthy way" all of the time, health promotion/wellness programs attempt to help change behavior and lifestyle in order to reduce the risk of various diseases and conditions. Logically, this method could be an effective answer to rising health care costs, but it is one of the most difficult to achieve.

What Are Health Promotion Programs?

Health promotion programs are a combination of education, activity and intervention to facilitate and reinforce a healthy lifestyle. Their purpose is to enhance worker job satisfaction and reduce the costs associated with accidents, absenteeism, lower productivity and health care. Such programs are defined and designed differently from organization to organization. The most common programs include worksite hypertension programs, smoking cessation, stress management, wellness and fitness programs, and nutrition and weight control programs.

Overall, there has been an increase in worksite health promotion activities since 1985. Which organizations tend to offer worksite wellness/health promotion programs? Approximately half of midsize to large companies offer such programs. Logically, large (more than 3,000 employees) companies are more likely than smaller companies to have a wellness program in place. The most popular type of program offered is basic screening for blood pressure and cholesterol. In order of diminishing proportion, other programs offered include educational newsletters on nutrition, healthy lifestyles and related topics; smoking cessation; weight loss programs; cancer screening; health club discounts/onsite health club facilities; and prenatal screening. The following are some examples of wellness/health promotion programs.

Worksite Hypertension Programs

Hypertension is often called the silent killer. It can go undetected for years, and most individuals with mild hypertension have no symptoms at all. Often there are no warning signs until the condition is advanced. When high blood pressure is uncontrolled for long periods, the heart, brain, kidneys and arteries become the major targets for damage. Although debate still rages about the strength of association among diet, smoking, obesity, excessive salt intake and hypertension, these factors have been shown to lead to high blood pressure. Not surprisingly, those with high blood pressure will be told to (1) lose weight, (2) restrict salt intake, (3) stop smoking and (4) start exercising.

Although one of the leading health conditions, affecting millions of Americans, high blood pressure is one of the most treatable and controllable; sharp reductions in the number of premature deaths and in cardiovascular diseases have been noted among those being treated. Antihypertensive drug therapy is often prescribed in combination with the above dictates, but the long-term effects of drug therapy, especially among those with mild hypertensive disease, are controversial. Consideration of the individual's risk factors, medical history and behavioral factors (including the likely compliance with therapy) will offer the best guidelines for the type of treatment plan.

The reason so many companies favor hypertension screening programs reflects the importance of identifying individuals with high blood pressure. Hypertension screening programs have been a popular and effective means of identifying those with high blood pressure and serve as an excellent conduit for evaluation and treatment.

Blood pressure screening is easy to do, but the sponsor must have a plan—a followup—to deal with those in need of treatment. The most basic of programs is purely educational in which information is made widely available. The costs associated with this approach are low, but the payoff is probably low too.

The next stage would be not only to educate the workforce, but also have a mechanism for screening whereby employees with elevated pressure would be encouraged to seek medical care. The costs associated with this type of program are modest, and the payoff could be modest to substantial.

Under a worksite detection and treatment type program, nurses serve as gatekeepers and refer employees to physicians for evaluation and treatment. Once a treatment plan is agreed upon, medication can be dispensed at the worksite and periodic monitoring by the nurses can ensure that the individual's blood pressure is under control. The dropout rate is much lower with this type of intervention. Because there is more followup contact, especially in the first year of treatment, the initial costs are higher. Studies have shown, however, that reduction in blood pressure can be greater in the more intensive worksite program and concomitant costs can be reduced.

Since drug therapy is the main therapeutic intervention for hypertension, drug costs associated with each type of program are of interest. Medication should be purchased wholesale to obtain maximum savings.

In summary, hypertension screening and treatment at the worksite can yield substantial savings and enhance the health and well-being of the employee. Available evidence indicates that the cost of caring for an average hypertensive patient in a worksite setting is well below the cost of care provided in a more traditional setting (physician's office or outpatient department).

Smoking Cessation

That smoking is a costly habit (costly in terms of an individual's health and in terms of actual dollars spent for medical care among smokers) is a gross understatement. If an organization decides to establish only one worksite health promotion program, smoking cessation should be the program of choice. The evidence is clear and overwhelming that cigarette smoke contaminates and pollutes the air and creates a health hazard not only to the smoker, but to all those around who rely on the same air supply. Cigarette smoking is the single behavior responsible for the most preventable deaths in society. The largest numbers of excess deaths among cigarette smokers are due to coronary heart disease, lung cancer and chronic obstructive lung disease. Clearly, the risk of death from lung cancer and morbidity due to bronchitis and emphysema increase with the number of cigarettes smoked, the duration of smoking, the tar and nicotine content of the cigarette, whether the smoker inhales and how young the individual was when he or she started to smoke.

Happily, the proportion of individuals who smoke has declined since the 1964 publication of the surgeon general's report. Unhappily, the incidence of smokers has increased the most among young women.

Common sense dictates that it is in the employer's best interest to do something about smoking in the workplace. In addition to instituting a "no smoking in the building" policy, most companies offer smoking cessation programs to help smokers kick the habit. These programs range from simple distribution of self-help materials to full-blown programs including behavior modification, positive reinforcement, support groups and the like. Strategies vary depending on the number of employees, the amount of funds allocated to the programs and the company's philosophy. Logically, the effectiveness of worksite smoking cessation interventions would be enhanced by promoting worksite norms supportive of nonsmoking.

Although it is difficult to calculate the long-term costs and benefits of smoking cessation programs, it would appear that any reduction in the number of employees who smoke would be beneficial. A prevention strategy that cuts down smoking could significantly reduce illness and improve health status; decreased smoking should result in a drop in respiratory infections, subsequent heart conditions and cancers. The potential savings are tremendous.

Stress Management

As we approach the 21st century, stress seems to be one of the most common complaints among individuals of all walks of life. Common symptoms include anxiety, depression, absenteeism and low morale. Most have difficulty concentrating and have a loss of interest in work. Undue stress is now known to undermine the functioning of the immune system and render individuals more susceptible to all kinds of ailments. In fact, it is estimated that 60-90% of all visits to health professionals are for some sort of stress-related disorder: cardiovascular disease, gastrointestinal disorders, tension and vascular headaches, lower back pain and depression. The direct and indirect costs associated with stress are extremely high.

Stress-related problems contribute to decreased production on the job causing workers to miss an average of 16 days each year. If, for example, productivity is dependent on the physical and psychological well-being of the individual, if this well-being is dependent on stress reduction and if stress and bad habits can be managed, then a fundamental change in the worker's health could have an enormous effect on productivity and the staggering amount of money lost due to poor productivity and lost work time.

Major sources of stress include:
- Personal—poor self-esteem, poor interpersonal communication, disruptive relationships, monetary problems, burnout/boredom, substance abuse, poor coping skills
- Environmental—job hazards/risks, job demands, poorly ergonomically designed work stations
- Organizational—role conflict, role ambiguity, management style, lack of control.

The 1990s saw an increase in a new form of stress: repetitive stress or repetitive trauma. Cumulative stress disorders have quadrupled in the last ten years and cost businesses over $20 billion annually! Repetitive stress accounts for 60% of all occupational injuries and the numbers continue to increase. Clearly, workplace ergonomic standards are needed to help reduce this rise.

Since stress is considered to be the nation's fastest growing occupational disease, it is not surprising that stress management programs are among the frequently offered worksite health promotion programs. The types of these programs include:

- Building awareness through education
- Assessment—focusing on individual stress assessment inventories
- Skills building—workshops to include relaxation skills, coping skills, interpersonal skills
- Therapeutic counseling
- Organizational and environmental changes in the workplace.

Are these programs successful? Are they cost-effective? Do they work over the long term? The results are spotty. Most stress management programs provide education about the sources of stress but do little to reduce work stressors. No study has looked at the long-term consequences of such programs. In the short term, however, a stress management program's greatest potential may be in lowering accident risk and subsequent insurance losses through a reduction of stress symptoms at the workplace.

Are these programs being utilized? Most wellness program sponsors use the level of employee participation as a measure of interest. If the program is not being utilized, if there is not a demonstrable change in employee behavior or decrease in sick days taken, for example, it is most likely that the program is not having an effect or achieving its goals.

Fitness Programs

Studies have shown that physical activity is inversely associated with morbidity and mortality from many chronic diseases. An increased level of physical fitness appears to be beneficial, primarily due to lowered rates of cardiovascular diseases and cancer. The data suggest that even a modest improvement in fitness level among the most unfit confers a substantial health benefit. That is, lower intensity activities, such as walking, can have benefits. Many organizations encourage their employees to walk during their lunch hour. Others with a more sophisticated workout arrangement encourage employees to utilize the facility, with some paying for club memberships. Regardless of the intensity of the fitness program, encouragement or incentives to exercise regularly should be part of the organization's culture.

Nutrition and Weight Control Programs

The role of dietary patterns and practices in preventing disease cannot be minimized. Overweight remains a national concern: Among adults age 20-74 years, the prevalence of those above the recommended weight level increased from 26% in 1976-1980 to 34% in 1988-1991. Among women age 20-34 years, overweight prevalence increased by 49% during this time period and among men age 55-64 years there was a 42% increase. Among males age 65-74 years during this same time period, there was a staggering 70% increase in the prevalence of overweight. Being overweight is a risk factor for diabetes, heart disease and hypertension. Adding to the misery, as anyone who has lost weight and then tried to keep it off can tell you, within five years the majority regain the weight that was lost. Studies have documented a metabolic and physiologic explanation for this high failure rate; however, a simple change in diet, one that is more nutritious in composition, can help enhance the health and well-being of the individual.

Since employees eat at least one main meal, as well as snacks, at the workplace, businesses have an excellent opportunity to affect the diet and food composition of their workforce. While it may not be possible to eliminate all nonnutritious foods from the diet at the worksite, a more sensible selection of foods can be provided. For example, healthful daily specials can be offered and foods very high in cholesterol and fats can be reduced. A daily listing indicating calories, cholesterol, fats and sodium content would help individuals in their effort to diet. An added side benefit might be the influence of healthful eating patterns in the home.

Some organizations provide employees with the opportunity to join a private weight reduction program. For those who manage to lose their desired number of pounds and to keep their weight down for a specified period of time, the company could offer to pay the membership fee or award a bonus. Since it takes great effort to keep those unwanted pounds off, any help the company can provide would be significant in the long term.

Do nutrition programs save money? The best answer is that the savings are immeasurable due to the potential benefits of a healthier employee. These programs should not be established primarily for cost-containment purposes; rather, they can help individuals become more conscious of eating well and nutritiously.

Other Options and Examples

Other worksite intervention programs are more educational than interventional. Health promotion/awareness events are typical of such programs. Injury prevention workshops are very important and attendance by all should be required. There are numerous newsletters, seminars, books, tapes and specialty organizations from which one could choose to get an idea of the types of programs available.

In the era of corporate downsizing and tight budgets, there are low-cost ways to promote corporate wellness. Self-care provides workers with information on self-management and is inexpensive yet supposedly effective. Individuals who have access to medical self-care resources have a lower perceived need for professional services as well as an increased appreciation for their own ability to help themselves. There are those who believe that employee health education and self-care in the form of personal learning experiences to improve health and decision making will have a substantial impact on health care costs in the short term. The data are not available on a large scale to affirm or refute this statement. In summary, each organization will have to make decisions based on its own philosophy, needs and wants. There is no shortage of health letters, newsletters and how-to seminars to help one choose!

Are Wellness Programs Cost-Effective?

Do these programs work and are they worth it? Answers, unfortunately are not easily come by. Indeed, the jury is still out as to whether or not the value of wellness programs are worth the cost. While some companies report lowered health care costs, reduced absenteeism and increased productivity, this author has seen little significant evidence to support such statements. There are so many confounding factors, which make it more difficult to draw conclusions.

Basically, the real worth and appeal of such programs is that they enhance and support corporate objectives and contribute to an environment that encourages a happy, healthy workforce. While cost is an important factor, the value of such programs often transcends economics. The bottom line may not be the most accurate way to assess the benefits of such programs. Indeed, increasing productivity and employee health and well-being may emerge as the real benefit rather than absolute cost savings.

Action Plan

Essentially, before any decision is made regarding the feasibility of establishing a health promotion/wellness program, there are several rules of thumb that should be followed:
- There must be labor, management and employee cooperation and participation in the program design.
- Assess the needs by reviewing claims and by paying attention to the demographics of the workforce.

- Decide on the type of intervention strategy—an educational program, evaluation screening, behavior support program.
- The needs of individual worksites must be considered. Employees need to see that the program is helpful and that it is in their best interest. Build a communication program around these tenets.
- Target goals. Have an evaluation plan ready so you can see if the program is working. Rely on feedback to gauge employee satisfaction and utilization.
- Address stressful working conditions.
- Decide how much you can afford to spend. Be sure to take into account long-term factors, not just short-term costs or savings.

Conclusion

In order for any organization to get a better handle on the health and well-being of its employees, health promotion should be encouraged. Since resources are scarce, programs that will give the best possible rate of return should be elected. Focus on smoking cessation, focus on easing stress in the workplace and focus on providing nutritious foods at the worksite. While no one activity, food or attitude can guarantee an illness-free ride to old age, the surest path to a better life is from a combination of factors including diet, exercise and stress management and the avoidance of health-robbing habits such as smoking, excessive drinking and poor diet. Changing one's lifestyle does have the potential to be a major factor to contain health care costs.

CHAPTER 7

The Costs of Substance Abuse

I t is commonly acknowledged that all forms of substance abuse and all forms of emotional and stress-related problems (personal, financial, mental, family) have a profound effect on the individual and on society. The medical, psychological, social and economic consequences of substance abuse can be devastating not only to the individual who is abusing alcohol or drugs, but also to those who interact with the abuser. To compound problems, the failure rate of detoxification and rehabilitation programs is high. If treatment could end the user's craving, as an injection of penicillin cures syphilis, addiction would be only a minor medical problem. Unfortunately, the social and personal problems resulting from addiction are notoriously difficult to deal with.

Not surprisingly, employers define the problem of substance abuse differently, and their views significantly determine the nature and scope of the organization's policies. While the majority of CEOs of Fortune 500 companies believe that drugs and alcohol are a problem in America, only 27% thought that their company had a problem. This head-in-the-sand approach could prove to be costly. Substance abuse has been shown to be a major problem in business and it is not limited to the clerical or lower management staff; many CEOs have sought treatment for their addiction. There is no glass ceiling for this problem.

This chapter focuses primarily on drug and alcohol abuse. The recurrent theme is that any form of substance abuse is a major problem in the workforce and represents an immense cost to the employer and to society. While the purpose is not to delve into the psychological aspects of addiction, this chapter will highlight the extent of substance abuse problems among the workforce, provide estimates of the costs of substance abuse and make the reader aware of the need for cost-containment options. The direct and indirect costs are substantial, and the employer's ability to manage these costs is difficult.

Who Is an Abuser?

Individuals with an addictive disorder use alcohol and/or other drugs compulsively even though most are aware of the potential for terrible consequences. Some drugs are highly addictive while others can be used for years before biochemical and/or physiological changes occur. For purposes herein, *substance abuse* refers to patterns of use lasting at least a month, which result in health consequences or impairment in social, psychological and occupational functioning. While it is difficult to predict who will develop a drug or alcohol habit, in general the situation becomes more serious when an individual becomes dependent. *Dependence* is characterized by compulsive use, craving and increased tolerance. There is compelling preoccupation with and loss of control over the substance. For someone to be considered an addict, he or she must develop a tolerance for the drug, be it alcohol or some other substance. That is, repeating the same dose causes a diminishing response and the drug leads to physical dependence. Repeated doses in greater quantities are needed to prevent pains of withdrawal.

The process of becoming dependent is complex and many factors play a role: the addictive properties of the drug(s), personality and existing psychiatric/psychological disorders, genetics and peer influence. It must be noted that the majority of those who drink or take illicit drugs do not experience problems. With heavier and more frequent consumption, however, the individual is more likely to experience problems with health, work, family members or the law.

According to the above definition, cocaine is not addictive per se, but alcohol and heroin are. This author will consider cocaine to be psychologically addictive; i.e., it is severely habit forming and it has the potential to induce a profound psychological dependence. From a medical standpoint, prolonged use of cocaine can cause severe psychological disturbances, and overdose results in collapse, convulsion and even death. Its abuse is a serious problem among the working population.

It should be stressed that the stereotype of a substance abuser living in an urban slum is hardly accurate. Abuse is not predominantly a minority problem either. All kinds of people in all kinds of places, those of both sexes and all lifestyles, abuse drugs and alcohol. Why do some become addicted when many are exposed to drugs? Do those who become addicted react differently to the drug, or do those who are not addicted have less need for gratification? Experts generally agree that there is no evidence that any one basic personality type is more susceptible than any other. Although the psychological factors that contribute to alcohol and drug abuse differ from individual to individual, the thesis maintained herein is that abuse should be dealt with like any other disease, and insurance coverage should be provided without prejudice or discrimination. The earlier the abuser can be detected and treated, the better the chance for success and the less costly the treatment will be in the long term.

Brief History

Today we are faced with an unprecedented array of substances produced in many parts of the world. An individual may sniff cocaine from Bolivia, inject heroin from Southeast Asia or may smoke marijuana from Jamaica and abuse diazepam manufactured in the United States. There are no global boundaries anymore.

As we approach the turn of another century, it is instructive to note that at this point in time 100 years ago there were virtually no restrictions on opiates, cocaine or marijuana. Individuals could obtain an assortment of drugs from mail-order catalogs, pharmacies and grocery stores. Marketing was unrestrained. Opium was valued for its soothing effects. Morphine was a popular painkiller, marijuana was used in cough preparations and cocaine was considered a miracle drug and touted as a cure for hay fever, syphilis and fatigue. Coca-Cola, as is now common knowledge, was the first to use cocaine in its syrup.

But, cocaine and heroin soon lost their luster as their addictiveness became apparent. Popular opinion began to view these drugs as a threat to the established social order. The Pure Food and Drug Act of 1906 required that packages and labels on medicines list any narcotic content. By requiring labeling, the act effectively destroyed the market for these substances. The Harrison Narcotics Act of 1914 imposed registration and recordkeeping requirements on the production and sale of opiates and cocaine. The Marijuana Tax Act of 1937 outlawed this substance. For decades thereafter, the laws prohibiting heroin, cocaine and marijuana have remained virtually unchanged. However, these laws have done little to reduce the supplies of illicit drugs or reduce the demand.

Since 1981, the federal government has spent more than $60 billion trying to curtail the drug trade (heroin, cocaine and marijuana). Despite this effort, drugs today are cheaper, more plentiful and purer than they were a decade ago. At the same time, the United States has the highest addiction rate in its history and (second to Russia) the highest rate of imprisonment in the world, largely due to drug-related crime.

Also, alcohol consumption in the United States has vacillated over the decades. Consumption was at its lowest during prohibition and the Depression years and the highest around the 1980s when more than half the states lowered the legal drinking age to 18. Alcohol consumption has declined recently primarily due to the raising of the minimum drinking age to 21 in all states.

The Extent of Substance Abuse

According to the National Household Survey, an amazing 24.4 million Americans (one in every eight) used illicit drugs in 1993, and half used drugs at least once a month. More than two-thirds of these regular users are employed. These figures do not include alcohol consumption, which is a legal substance.

It is estimated that in 1993, drug use increased for the first time in a decade, ending the trend in which cocaine and marijuana use had steadily declined. Although heroin use has remained fairly steady, the availability of cheaper and purer heroin, which is usually smoked or snorted rather than injected, has posed new dangers to users. Of those accustomed to weaker heroin, the risks of overdosing and, in some cases, dying have increased dramatically.

Most individuals who have a drinking problem, or who have developed alcohol dependence, are employed and have a family. In fact, most alcoholics work full time. Consider the following:

- Alcohol abuse is estimated to afflict over ten million people in the United States.
- Alcohol abuse, like drug abuse, recognizes no social boundaries nor is it restricted by education, economics, profession or gender.
- The cost of alcohol abuse is tremendous; over $60 billion a year is attributed to alcohol abuse.
- Alcohol-related problems cause thousands of deaths through alcoholic damage to the stomach, liver, heart, brain and immune system. The number of fatal highway accidents and industrial accidents continues to climb each year.

Alcoholism, the end product of severe alcohol abuse, is a progressive disease that is a treatable illness. The problem is that many alcoholics deny that they have a problem; a high percentage referred for care fail to follow through the full course of treatment; and, for those who do complete treatment, the recidivism rate is unfortunately high. Indeed, treatment outcomes often vary from alcoholic to alcoholic, depending on the individual's motivations; economic, personal and social supports; and job/home stability.

Cost Factors

The economics of substance abuse is staggering. The costs include emergency room medical care; the expense of treating the abuser's addiction in treatment facilities; productivity losses caused by premature disability or death; and costs related to crime, destruction of property, and other losses. Applying a dollar figure is difficult because of the differences in calculations, but estimates imply that almost $99 billion is attributed to alcohol abuse and $67 billion to illicit drug abuse. The costs of these substances related significantly to productivity losses associated with death and illness.

In addition to the costs of drug/alcohol-related workplace injuries, the health insurance costs for employees with drug/alcohol problems are twice those of other employees. The 1991 National Household Survey on Drug Abuse found that over one-quarter of full-time employed illicit drug users reported that they had missed work due to illness or injury in the past 30 days, and 18% simply skipped work. Fifteen percent admitted being high or drunk while on the job and 10% missed work due to their problem. Figure 1 shows the extent of alcohol and drug users' problems working.

A study by the Center on Addiction and Substance Abuse at Columbia University estimated that in fiscal year 1995, substance abuse and addiction accounted for $77.6 billion in federal entitlement payments, or nearly 20% of the total that the federal government will spend on these programs in that year. Almost 90% of this figure constitutes health care and disability costs stemming from substance abuse (tobacco representing the largest part of the $66.4 billion).

Treatment is the most effective way to reduce the personal and economic costs of addiction as compared to other methods. Figure 2 clearly shows that treatment for cocaine use, for example, is far more cost-effective than domestic enforcement, interdiction or source country control. According to the National Institute on Drug Abuse, each dollar spent on treatment saves between $4 and $7 in reduced costs to the public and adds $3 in increased

FIGURE 1

Alcohol and Drug Users Have Problems Working, 1991

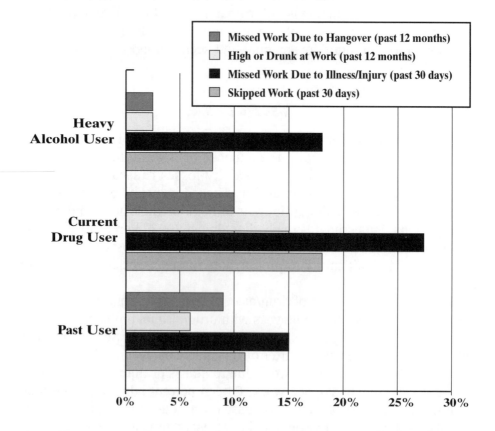

Legend:
- Missed Work Due to Hangover (past 12 months)
- High or Drunk at Work (past 12 months)
- Missed Work Due to Illness/Injury (past 30 days)
- Skipped Work (past 30 days)

Categories: Heavy Alcohol User, Current Drug User, Past User

Source: 1991 *National Household Survey on Drug Abuse.* U.S. Substance Abuse and Mental Health Services Administration.

productivity. A 1994 California study found that $1 invested in alcohol and drug treatment programs saved $7.14 in future costs, and the Rand Corporation reported that providing treatment for addicts would save more than $150 billion in social costs over the next 15 years. The Small Business Administration reported that drug-free workplace programs produced a significant return on investment because of reduced employee turnover and increased productivity. Workplace programs cost anywhere between $22 and $50 per employee, but it costs an estimated $640 in annual workforce costs incurred by each untreated drug abuser.

FIGURE 2

Treatment Is Most Cost-Effective Way to Cut Drug Use
Cost of Reducing Cocaine Consumption by 1% (in millions per year)

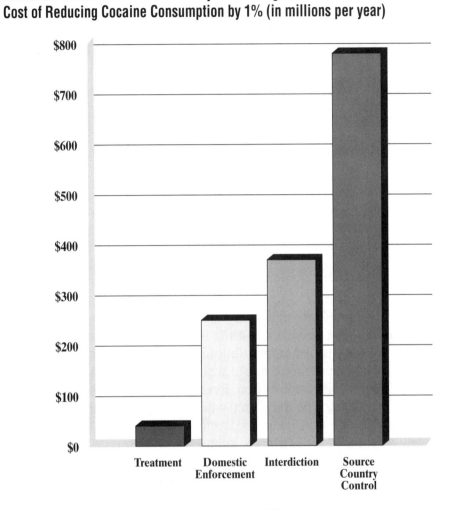

Source: RAND Drug Policy Research Center, Santa Monica, California.

Dealing With Substance Abuse at the Workplace

It was the cocaine epidemic of the 1980s that served to galvanize business to begin to understand and address how pervasive drugs were in the workplace. Indeed, drug abuse was not then, nor is now, a rare occurrence. More than two-thirds of regular users are employed and 15% admitted to going to work while under the influence. As such, in 1986 President Reagan issued an executive order which required that all federal employees refrain from using illicit drugs on or off the job. The goal of this order was to establish or foster a drug-free federal workplace. More recently, federal requirements mandated that government contractors and grantees receiving more than $25,000 in federal funds have a drug-free workplace policy that includes sanctions for drug use. The Employee Testing Act of 1991 required alcohol testing for the first time.

Following the government's lead, nonfederal employers, too, affirmed that employees who abuse alcohol or drugs must be evaluated and either treated or removed from the workplace. Realistically, however, economics provided the impetus rather than any altruistic feelings. Illicit drug and alcohol abuse are costly to the employer. Employed drug abusers as compared to their nonabusing counterparts are:

- Three times more likely to be late for work
- Ten times as likely to miss work
- 3.6 times more likely to injure themselves or another person in a workplace accident and are responsible for 40% of all industrial fatalities
- Five times more likely to file a workers' compensation claim
- 33% less productive
- Likely to incur 300% higher medical costs and benefits.

It is important to remember that the last thing a substance abuser is willing to sacrifice is his or her job. Not only is the job the major source of income (particularly necessary if one is sustaining a cocaine habit), but it is also a symbol of the ability to function. Even though the illness may be blatantly obvious to others, the individual's denial of reality makes it difficult to convince the abuser that he or she needs help. In particular, substance abusers will accept the loss of friends, spouses and children without changing their habits. The threat of job loss, however, is one of the most effective means of motivating these individuals to seek treatment.

The importance of the work environment in providing the substance abuser with the means and motivation to stop cannot be emphasized enough. The threat of being fired from the work environment has a powerful influence on drinking and drug abuse behavior and, as such, can reinforce the necessity for the individual to seek treatment. Confronting the abuser about the serious consequences of his or her behavior can serve to maximize the effectiveness of treatment. Although an employer cannot force an abuser to seek help, the individual must be sufficiently motivated to deal with his or her drug/alcohol problem.

What are the employer's options? How should employers respond? What are the legal limitations? Should random drug testing at the workplace be implemented? Should pre-employment testing be implemented? What kind of employee assistance programs (EAPs) should be established? These issues will be discussed in greater detail subsequently.

Evolution of Substance Abuse Treatment Programs

There was a rapid expansion in drug and alcohol treatment programs during the 1960s and 1970s. During this time period, there was a recognition that substance abuse disorders should be considered diseases, which was a major step for treatment to be reimbursable. Whereas the treatment systems in the 1970s were generated by heroin addiction, the growth in the 1980s was a result of the millions who developed cocaine, alcohol and marijuana problems. Private rehabilitation programs, chemical dependency units in psychiatric and general hospitals, and specialized private practitioners proliferated to treat the growing addict population, many of whom were often middle class or affluent.

The 1980s and 1990s witnessed a decrease in the number of programs primarily because insurance companies and managed care organizations became more rigorous in denying various treatment modalities, reducing length of stay and reducing reimbursable costs. Unfortunately, this action came at a time when the demand for treatment was at its highest. It is this author's belief that cutting benefits is not likely to be cost-effective in the long term. Such action often leads to delayed treatment and, ultimately, higher costs. It is far more sensible to develop a rational substance abuse policy with cost-containment features.

The importance of the work environment in providing the abuser with the means and motivation to seek treatment must be underscored. Extensive research has shown that:

- Prevention and treatment can substantially reduce the demand for drugs.
- Drug testing combined with treatment can reduce employee drug use and improve productivity and safety.
- Aftercare and/or self-help groups, such as Alcoholics Anonymous or Narcotics Anonymous, are more likely to help the recovering addict to remain abstinent. The longer the individual attends such a group, the greater the likelihood that he or she will remain drug free.

Principles of Effective Treatment

Substance abuse treatment can be effective and can decrease the use of alcohol and drugs. For some individuals, a brief intervention can be effective, while others will require more intensive services and sometimes repeat treatment interventions. The key to an effective treatment program is to match the individual with the intervention most appropriate for him or her. Figures 3A and 3B show the type of treatment interventions as well as the principal drugs used by the individuals in treatment. After alcohol, the primary drug of abuse is cocaine or its derivative crack, followed by heroin and other opiates. (Poly-drug use is most common among those in treatment.) Almost all are in outpatient programs, documenting the trend away from inpatient care.

Substance abuse treatment takes many forms; and, although there is no one typical type of program, most can be loosely grouped into one or more of the following:

- Detoxification: The purpose is the therapeutic, supervised withdrawal from the intoxicating effects of alcohol or other drugs. It is an important first step in the treatment process, but has little lasting impact in and of itself.
- Residential programs: These are highly structured programs either short term (two to four weeks) or therapeutic communities (TCs). The former focus on educating patients about the effects of alcohol and other drugs, teaching life skills and stress management, providing therapy and encouraging lifestyle changes. The latter are drug-free programs set in nonmedical, community facilities in which patients spend more than six months progressing through a hierarchy of treatment modalities.
- Outpatient programs: Focus is on intensive day treatment in which the patient attends group counseling, individual therapy, skills development and educational/vocational training for four to eight hours every day for three to six months, or less intensive outpatient programs offering similar services once or twice a week from three to six months. Continuing care is less formal relapse prevention and could continue for years. Focus is on self-help, group meetings and peer interactions.

To recover from an addiction, an individual needs to develop new patterns of living, new coping skills and new support networks. Without these factors, relapse is almost guaranteed. Finding the right type of program for the addict is crucial. For those with a heroin addiction, treatment generally focuses on opioid substitution therapy, which blocks the craving for heroin and keeps the individual healthy during heroin withdrawal. Currently, three medications are approved for such use: methadone, naltrexone and levo-alpha-acetyl methadol. These drugs are only effective in treating heroin and other opiate addiction. To succeed, opioid substitution must be offered in conjunction with medical, counseling and rehabilitation services.

FIGURE 3A

Clients in Alcohol or Drug Specialty Treatment: 1991

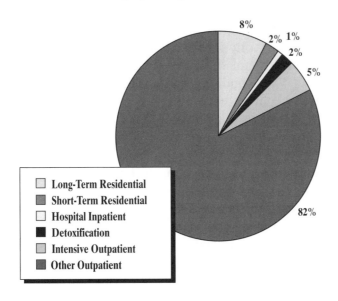

☐ Long-Term Residential
■ Short-Term Residential
☐ Hospital Inpatient
■ Detoxification
☐ Intensive Outpatient
■ Other Outpatient

Source: U.S. Substance Abuse and Mental Health Services Administration.

FIGURE 3B

Principal Drugs Used by Clients in Specialty Treatment: 1990

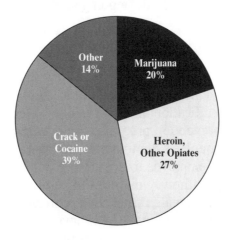

Source: U.S. National Institute on Drug Abuse/1990 Drug Services Research Survey.

The Costs of Substance Abuse _____ 115

Treatment for cocaine addiction is more difficult because there is no substitution therapy for this substance. One of the most promising treatments is the neurobehavioral model in which the addict learns adaptive social and stress management skills. Counseling is imperative and random weekly urine tests will document abstinence/relapse.

Alcohol addiction is most often treated with detoxification and counseling, as well as by new treatment strategies such as:

- Aversion therapy (When conditioning is successful, alcohol will provoke an automatic negative response.)
- Behavioral self-control training (encourages the decrease in consumption and a reduction in the negative consequences of problem drinking)
- Marital and family therapy (in an effort to have the family support and encourage the problem drinker).

Since many with addictive disorders also have mental disorders and are poly-drug abusers, treatment must address all elements which led to the addiction. A combination of detoxification, inpatient and outpatient treatment, and aftercare programs is warranted. Regardless of the type of treatment program, several principles must be acknowledged:

- The program must provide for a continuum of care and comprehensive coordinated services.
- The program must equip the addict with psychosocial rehabilitation (life skills, coping, etc.).
- The program must be highly structured and provide intensive individualized attention and pair the addict with the combination of services best suited to him or her.
- The program should provide ongoing staff development and training.

Basic Components of Workplace Programs

The primary components of any worksite substance abuse program should include a prevention and educational component as well as the provision for early identification and treatment or referral. Many companies have instituted drug prevention programs and awareness training to teach supervisors how to recognize symptoms of alcohol and drug abuse. The employer should help the employee to ensure the quality of work and to enhance worksite safety without violating the employee's privacy. Effective programs can be compassionate rather than coercive or harsh.

Employee assistance programs (EAPs) have been established to address the growing incidence of substance abuse at the workplace. The philosophy behind the concept is that the employee can be helped (treated and rehabilitated) at the point when the abuse of alcohol and/or drugs has not yet progressed to a more advanced (and more costly) stage. The motivating force is to contain the high costs of substance abuse and return the worker to the workforce.

There is no right way to establish an EAP. Any good program, however, must include prevention, treatment and rehabilitation. It must be viewed as being nonpunitive, nonjudgmental and confidential. A successful EAP must also incorporate various strategies to address the crucial issue of denial. Since substance abusers are very good at manipulating others, the strategy of *constructive confrontation* (i.e., meeting face to face with the employee to confront him or her with facts about the problem) is effective in addressing the psychodynamics that usually accompany abuse. In a context of constructive confrontation, help is offered and, at the same time, it is made clear that job penalties or job loss will be considered if help is not accepted or if performance continues to deteriorate.

One of the greatest potential problems of this technique is getting supervisors to identify and confront subordinates in need of treatment. When supervisors are reluctant to become involved, it should be made clear to them that substance abuse is to be treated sympathetically without threatening employment status. A supervisor's intervention is not only permissible, but strongly encouraged. The supervisor is not betraying anyone; he or she, based on poor job performance indicators, is merely referring the employee to those competent to diagnose the problem and institute appropriate therapy.

Every company should have a written policy regarding their EAP. Included in the policy should be the following:

- Alcohol and drug abuse are treatable medical problems.
- Those employees who are performing oddly or poorly will be confronted; and constructive, positive support for treatment and rehabilitation will be offered in a confidential manner.
- If an employee's performance does not improve, the company will take disciplinary measures.
- Top management and union hierarchy must fully support the aims and objectives of the program. Management must not only be familiar with the program, but also must support it. Little familiarity, meager program resources and lack of formally designated program personnel can effectively render an EAP impotent. Cooperation is required by all levels of management as well as by the rank and file.
- The program is to be available to all employees at all levels; substance abuse is as common in the factory as it is in the boardroom.

A company can establish its own in-house EAP or can contract with an outside firm specializing in treatment and rehabilitation. In-house EAPs should be staffed by trained personnel. There are, however, significant startup costs and, because of concerns about confidentiality, such programs often require more time to gain employee trust and subsequent utilization. In-house programs should also offer educational lectures, self-help groups and family involvement, in addition to group and individual counseling. Independent firms can be retained to administer the EAP. In fact, treating substance abuse for profit has become one of the fastest growing markets in the health care field.

While most large employers have a workplace drug policy, small companies can and should develop one as well. The National Drugs Don't Work Partnership is an organization that brings employers together to eliminate drugs and alcohol from their workplaces; it focuses on helping businesses with 20-1,000 employees, and has presently attracted more than 400 such businesses to its cause.

Do EAPs Work?

The question of whether EAPs work is often difficult to discern. Methodologies differ, outcome factors may not be similar, the focus may differ making generalizations difficult. Most EAPs show initially high costs; some do realize long-term savings. A government report assessing the effectiveness of substance abuse treatment programs has compiled a listing of successful programs and is an excellent resource. In general, successful programs are guided by a well-articulated philosophy; have a highly trained staff; conduct continuous, detailed client assessments; develop individualized treatment plans; and offer continuing care. They also offer or directly link clients to a full spectrum of health, education and social services to equip individuals to function productively after treatment.

Every EAP should be evaluated to ascertain whether the program is working as intended and how many employees have been seen, with what problems, for how long and by whom. How much did the treatment cost? How effective has the treatment been over the long term? Who is monitoring the services delivered to the employees? Success should not be limited to assessing the progress made by those in the program. Rather, it should include some measure of how many are being identified as in need and referred for help. If it is estimated that 6% of employees need assistance and only 1% are being referred, the program is obviously not working as intended. Finding out the degree of success in rehabilitation efforts and in identifying areas for program improvement can be facilitated by knowing the following:
- Sources of referral
- Demographic information about program clients
- Number of successful rehabilitations, according to your definition

- Estimates of job efficiency (compared to before treatment performance)
- Reduction in absenteeism, accidents and disability insurance benefits.

Drug Testing at the Workplace

One of the most controversial issues confronting employers is whether to test for substance use at the workplace. Although the federal government provides very little guidance for policy implementation and not enough funding to help the private sector to start drug testing and/or employee assistance programs, over eight in ten American companies now perform some type of drug testing among prospective or current employees. Drug testing of job applicants is by far the most widespread type of screening. Pre-employment testing has proved to be effective in screening out applicants who use drugs. Clearly, as this type of testing becomes common practice, the pressure will build on nontesting organizations to protect themselves against applicants who are not able to pass a drug test.

Random testing, that is, the testing of employees without advance warning, is by far the most controversial use of drug testing. Legal challenges (most of which assert that random testing violates an employee's rights to privacy) deter many organizations from instituting such a policy. One way to avoid charges of discrimination is to institute universal random testing to test all employees from the CEO down. The federal government, for example, does require random testing of workers whose jobs affect public health, safety and national security.

From a legal perspective, drug testing programs can be used to protect employee health and safety and enforce legitimate work performance standards, but only if they do so without violating the individual rights of employees. Employers should also evaluate the need for such a program. Another consideration is whom to test: job applicants, current employees, both? The courts have found pre-employment testing acceptable as long as it is consistent and nondiscriminatory. The success of a drug testing program depends on the program's commitment to confidentiality, rehabilitation, fairness and enforcement of work standards. By informing employees about all aspects of a drug testing program, employers can help circumvent future legal problems.

How an employer decides to handle employees found using drugs must be elucidated in the company's written policy. It must be explained clearly just what the company's position is regarding the use of drugs and alcohol at the workplace and the disciplinary measures that will be taken if an employee is found abusing any substance, working under the influence or possessing any substance.

Written Policy Should Be Reviewed by Legal Counsel

Since 1987, drug testing in major American companies has increased by more than 300%. According to an American Management Association survey, random drug testing in conjunction with education, training, counseling and treatment have a measurable effect on reducing drug use. Data clearly show that the percentage of workers testing positive has steadily declined. Perhaps awareness that a company may test for drugs has discouraged substance users from continuing their habit. In fact, the policy has served to encourage many to report their alcohol or drug problem in order to obtain help. There is a direct year-to-year correlation between the increase in random or periodic testing and the decrease in positive test rates. Figure 4 shows the trend in positive drug tests. Drug testing is strongly supported by the public.

Summary

Any effort to reduce drug abuse must recognize the central importance of the workplace. Employment is a powerful incentive to get help for one's addiction; the last thing an addict is willing to sacrifice is his or her job. Since the majority of addicts are currently employed, all employers—large and small—should establish a comprehensive, drug-free program. EAPs are viewed as an excellent means of providing confidential assistance with substance abuse as well as with personal problems. They have helped rehabilitate employees, thus reducing the costs associated with alcohol and drug use. But, each employer must decide on the nature and scope of its program based on an evaluation of the extent of the problem, the amount of money being expended for mental health claims, and estimates of lost productivity and absenteeism. Regardless of the type of program or policy, there must be support from all levels of management.

With substance abuse such a serious problem in the workplace, each organization must consider what they are (or are not) doing about managing these costs better. The information cited in this chapter should have made it clear that substance abuse among the workforce, in terms of lost productivity, absenteeism, accidents, medical claims and thefts, costs billions of dollars. Under the circumstances, employers have a strong economic motive for reducing employee substance abuse.

While businesses have chosen different approaches to address the use of drugs in the workplace, effective workplace programs, which provide confidential assistance for employees with substance abuse problems, do pay off as those organizations adapting a strong antidrug program show a reduction in absenteeism and employee turnover, and substantial decline in

FIGURE 4

Percentage of U.S. Workers Testing Positive for Drugs: 1988-1994

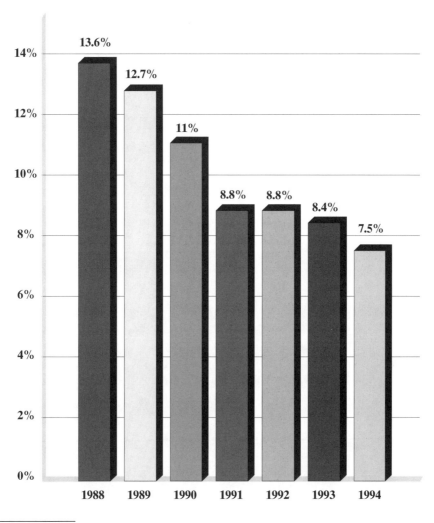

Source: SmithKline Beecham Clinical Laboratories, 1995.

positive drug tests among new applicants. When employees know that their jobs depend on their coming to work drug free, and when they know that their employer will help them kick their habit, they are much more likely to succeed in giving up drugs and alcohol. The economic and human costs are too high to ignore.

CHAPTER 8

Focus on Workers' Compensation

Workers' Compensation: Every state has a system providing employees who suffer job-related illnesses or injuries and to dependents of those killed in industry. Absolute liability is imposed on the employer, which is required to pay benefits prescribed by law.*

Industrial injury, occupational disease and workers' compensation have not been topics of headline caliber for many years. Although periodically a newsworthy industrial accident does make the front page of the newspapers, in general these issues have taken a back seat to health care reform. Within recent years, however, there has been more focus on workplace safety, job-related diseases and, in particular, the high costs of workers' compensation. As we approach the 21st century, there is a strong movement to address the cost issues associated with worksite injuries.

Hazards in the workplace include chemical, physical, biologic, ergonomic and socioemotional factors. Chemical hazards may appear as vapor, fumes,

---

*Employee Benefit Plans: A Glossary of Terms, 8th ed. (Brookfield, WI: International Foundation of Employee Benefit Plans, 1993).

mists, gases or dust, and routes of entry may be by inhalation, ingestion or absorption by the skin. Poorly ventilated areas, for example, are the prime suspect in illnesses arising from chemical exposure. Physical hazards include heat, cold, atmospheric pressure, light, radiation, vibration and noise. Biologic hazards include infectious agents, toxins/poisons, and insect and animal contamination. Ergonomic hazards result from poorly designed equipment for the operator's purposes, and socioemotional hazards encompass stress and the psychological impact on a worker's health. The latter two can result from worker fatigue, back/head/neck problems, tenosynovitis or other soft tissue inflammation.

Clearly, addressing potential hazards could do much to minimize accidents and illnesses at the workplace. Industrial hygienists and occupational health specialists are trained to monitor worksite safety. By identifying potential health hazards, recommendations for new health and safety programs or improved control efforts can be made.

Historical Background

As industries grew at the beginning of the 20th century, so did injuries associated with these industries. Stories of mutilations and death in factories and mines were quite common. At that time, for example, Upton Sinclair's expose of the meat packing industry eloquently exposed horrific conditions in slaughterhouses. Indeed, the period from 1903-1907 represents the highest industrial accident rate in U.S. history. Railroads alone were responsible for the deaths of 3,500 individuals, and this figure does not take into account those who were injured on the job. In response to the proliferation of job-related injuries (traumatic injury on the job occurred with monotonous regularity), public discontent with the manner in which job-related disabilities were handled provided the impetus for the enactment of workers' compensation laws. In fact, workers' compensation is the oldest social insurance program in the United States, dating from 1908-1911. Its purpose was to provide benefits to workers disabled from work-related injury or illness and to dependents of workers whose deaths resulted from such injury or illness. In return for employers assuming the costs of occupational disabilities, without regard to fault involved, employers were relieved of liability from common law suits involving negligence. The employee is not awarded money for nonspecific damages such as pain and suffering or emotional distress. Although the employee's financial recovery is much smaller than a tort recovery (for negligence), it is intended to be immediate, secure and less expensive for the employee to obtain. Hence, workers' compensation was set up to represent a compromise for employers and employees alike. That is, the employee will recover for *any* injury suffered in the course and scope of employment, regardless of fault, and the employer benefits by avoiding exposure for claims of punitive damages, bad faith or unfair claim settlement practices. Unlike health insurance, workers' compensation does not require a contribution from the employee—the employer pays the entire premium—and coverage is immediate and automatic. Table I highlights the differences between the two types of insurance.

By the early 1930s, most states had passed workers' compensation laws to protect workers, and today all 50 states have adopted some form of workers' compensation legislation. Although there are as many workers' compensation laws as there are state jurisdictions, there are general similarities among them. Workers' compensation laws are compulsory for employers with a minimum number of workers in all states except South Carolina, Texas and New Jersey. But, employers in these states face significant financial liability if like benefits are not provided.

Each jurisdiction has a commission or board to implement its workers' compensation act, and the members of these commissions are responsible for adjudicating cases. Their role is to determine whether an injury or illness is truly work related and to determine in dollar terms how a worker's injury or illness has affected the wage-earning capacity of the injured worker. The administrative law judges are final arbiters. Given the differences in composition of the commissions and the fact that the benefits are not scientifically determined, it is not surprising that discrepancies abound. Many injured workers seek assistance from attorneys to navigate the complex administrative maze and to bargain with insurance companies and employers for compensation. Attorneys increase awards in cases that go to arbitration, but their involvement increases the likelihood of a settlement and, in these cases, the payout is substantially lower than that for workers with similar cases who are not represented by attorneys.

Despite the enactment of workers' compensation laws, workplace safety continued to be of concern. Although Congress enacted comprehensive labor relations legislation in 1935 (National Labor Relations Act) and comprehensive wage and hour legislation in 1938 (Fair Labor Standards Act), it did not pass any comprehensive safety and health laws until 1970. The Occupational Safety and Health Act of 1970 (OSH Act) provided a regulatory vehicle for assuring worker safety and health. The act set standards of safety that would prevent injury and/or illness among workers. Congress finally took action, but only after years of public concern regarding workplace hazards. The impetus was testimony asserting that industry was not only hazardous but also costly in terms of the time lost from work due to injury or illness.

TABLE I

Workers' Compensation vs. Health Insurance

DEFINITION

Workers' compensation is a social contract between employer and employees that provides a no-fault solution for injuries and illnesses during employment. Employees give up the right to sue their employer in return for prompt and certain benefits. Each state specifies the benefits and how they are administered, and employers are subject to substantial penalties for failure to pay benefits.

Employer-provided health insurance originated during World War II and the era of wage controls. Fringe benefits, including medical care, were used to attract and retain an experienced workforce.

COMPULSORY VS. VOLUNTARY

A compulsory program that requires employers to ensure payment of benefits through the purchase of an insurance policy or self-insurance plan that is regulated by the state.

Voluntary on the employer's part except if included in a collective bargaining agreement. Employers purchase a policy or pay benefits without regulatory supervision. The form of insurance is at the employer's discretion and may involve a commercial carrier, prepaid plans, HMO, PPO or a combination of services.

SCOPE OF COVERAGE

Coverage is immediate and automatic, commencing with the first day of work. All types of employees are covered—regular, temporary, full time, part time, even illegally employed minors and aliens. Preexisting conditions are included.

Usually subject to a waiting period and preexisting conditions are excluded, at least during a specified treatment-free period. Coverage of part-time and seasonal employees may be limited or not available.

EXTENT OF COVERAGE

Operates on an occurrence basis. Once a job-related injury or illness occurs, the employee is covered for its consequences, even if the worker changes jobs or retires.

Extent of coverage treatment based, paying only for treatment provided while the coverage is in effect. There is no coverage if the employee switches jobs or if the employers change to a different insurer.

BENEFITS

Varies by state, but usually covers all reasonably required medical services to cure or relieve the effects of the injury. Has no time or amount limits and has a wage replacement component for the time the employee is unable to work because of the illness or injury. Includes vocational rehab services and additional payments if the injury results in permanent impairment, and payment to surviving dependents in the event of death.

Pays only for medical treatment and related services as specified in the contract. Subject to maximum limitations by year and employee lifetime. Disability payments, vocational rehab services and death benefits are not offered except as separate policies.

COST SHARING

Cost is borne entirely by the employer through an insurance carrier or employer is self-insured. No contributions by employees.

Employees usually pay a portion of the cost of insurance through deductibles, copayments, coinsurance, requirements and, frequently, part of the monthly premium.

RATE REGULATIONS

Regulated by individual state's insurance commission and pricing structure. Includes financial incentives for the safety-conscious employer.

Basically, no government regulation and health insurers may charge what the marketplace dictates or permits. Premium levels are community rated, and there are no guaranteed economic incentives, i.e., discounts if the employer (and employees) control or reduce costs.

Source: TCM 65: April/May/June 1994.

Included in the act are (1) health standards to protect workers from exposure to harmful physical or chemical agents in the workplace and (2) safety standards to protect against imminent physical "insults" such as falls, fires, construction collapse and the like. The act also requires a monitoring of the workplace and establishes exposure standards and guidelines designed to keep worker exposure to harmful agents below levels likely to have an adverse effect on health.

The Occupational Safety and Health Administration (OSHA) was created within the Department of Labor to administer the new law. OSHA is responsible for promulgating legally enforceable health and safety standards for among other things clean air, toxic substances, cancer causing chemicals, biological agents and radiation. Its mandate is to encourage employers and employees to reduce the number of workplace hazards and to institute new or improved safety and health programs; to authorize the secretary of labor to set mandatory occupational safety and health standards covering all businesses engaged in interstate commerce; to maintain a reporting and record-keeping system to monitor job-related injuries and illnesses; and to encourage joint labor-management efforts to reduce injury and disease arising out of employment.

In addition to the OHS Act and OSHA, the National Institute of Occupational Safety and Health (NIOSH) was created as an agency of the U.S. Public Health Service under the Centers for Disease Control and Prevention. NIOSH is responsible for conducting research about job safety and health hazards and for developing methods for protecting employees. NIOSH is not an enforcement agency but a research agency.

Whereas reform initially focused on the acute problem of traumatic *injury* rather than on *occupational disease,* over time the acknowledgment of health hazards that cause disease has shifted the focus to *disease prevention.*

What Triggers a Workers' Compensation Claim?

The vast majority of workers who sustain a work-related injury or illness only require medical treatment and experience little, if any, interruptions in their life or work. Most of these injuries never become workers' compensation cases because they are treated to the satisfaction of the company and the injured employee. It is the minority of cases for which a clear-cut cause and effect are not evident, for which a long-term rehabilitation is required, or for which the medical conditions may be partially related to work or partially related to other causes that sets the stage for a confrontation. In these cases, early, prompt investigation and documentation by the employer are recommended. When, where and how did the incident occur? Who was with the injured employee? What specific body parts were affected and what are the employee's symptoms?

It is generally accepted that any *worksite accident* (defined usually as unexpected, unintended and unforeseen events occurring at the workplace) or *occupationally related disease* (a condition resulting or stemming from employment) is compensable under the law. But an injured worker must prove that the injury or disease was sustained in the "course and scope of employment" for which a "due and timely notice" was given the employer. Medical causation must be shown to be work related. While emotional conditions arising out of employment or overlapping from work-related injuries are compensable, it must be proven that they were sustained in the course and scope of employment.

In all cases, the injury must be shown to have caused some functional impairment or disability; e.g., a harmful change in a human organism as a result of the work-related accident, condition or exposure as well as the degree to which the employee is functionally or occupationally impaired as a result of that "harmful change." In some jurisdictions, there must also be a diminished wage-earning capacity known as *occupational disability.* When a worker, for example, breaks a leg or an arm or suffers head trauma as a result of a fall at work, the issue of worksite injury is clear. With regard to back sprains, cumulative trauma injuries such as carpal tunnel syndrome, or emotional distress, however, the question of whether the injury is work related is often contested by the employer. Further complicating matters is the issue of preexisting conditions.

The percentage of impairment attributable to the preexisting condition is taken into account in the compensation award to the employee, and the employer is not responsible to pay this percentage. But, if the injury is preexisting and dormant and the worksite trauma activates or aggravates the condition, that percentage is paid for generally by a second injury or special fund (statewide funds). While preexisting conditions are taken into account, subsequent injuries are not considered.

As an example, John Doe suffers a heart attack at work. The question is, did the heart attack occur by coincidence or was it caused by a preexisting condition such as hypertension or arteriosclerosis? With regard to back cases, did Jane Smith's degenerative disk disease contribute to her sustaining the on-the-job back injury? Was Susan Jones' carpal tunnel syndrome a result of the repetitive motions required to do her job, or from the gardening and ironing she did at home? The employer may argue that it should not be responsible for that percentage of the injury caused by preexisting conditions or daily chores unrelated to work. The employee would counter that the disability would not be an issue *but for* the conditions at the workplace.

For those cases that are adjudicated by workers' compensation systems, there generally is a clear understanding of the nature of the medical condition and a clear relationship of that condition to some employment situation that caused it. While it is often easier to show cause for a work-related accident, work-related diseases are often more troublesome due to confounding factors and an often lengthy time needed to show cause and effect (epidemiologic studies take time; often the lead time from the time of exposure to the onset of disease is many years, complicating matters). There is a listing of illnesses that are known to be associated with specific industries. Black lung, for example, is a known ailment associated with exposure to coal dust; asbestosis is a known ailment associated with exposure to asbestos fibers; contact dermatitis is known to result from exposure to chemical irritants; and certain cancers are more common among oil workers. Yet, work-relatedness must still be established. Confounding nonoccupational factors such as age, sex and medical conditions such as arthritis and the like are often brought into the discussion.

Defining Disability

The classification of disability is generally made by a physician, who plays a pivotal role in deciding whether the injury or disease arises out of and in the course of employment—AOE/COE. Benefits are tailored to the nature of the disability and are based on the percentage of occupational impairment. Since disability benefits are intended to compensate an injured employee for the lost income sustained as a result of an on-the-job injury, classification of the disability becomes very important.

Unfortunately, there is no universally agreed-upon definition of *disability*. The American Medical Association's *Guides to the Evaluation of Permanent Impairment (Guides)* defines *disability* as a "decrease in or the loss or absence of the capacity of an individual to meet personal, social, or occupational demands, or to meet statutory or regulatory requirements." While vague in language, the *Guides* give the physician some guidance in determining the presence, nature and extent of a person's impairment or set of impairments. Based on the guidelines, the physician determines the percentage of permanent impairment, if any. The physician must also state whether the employee will be required to work under any restrictions in the future. This determination establishes the foundation for the disability benefits.

When the injured employee reaches maximum medical improvement, the issue of whether the individual has sustained a permanent impairment is critical. However, under workers' compensation, an impaired person may not receive benefits if an adjudicator determines that the impairments were not caused or aggravated by or did not arise out of employment. Generally, the determination of functional impairment focuses on "permanent partial disability" or "permanent total disability." The actual impairment is translated into a dollar amount pursuant to a specific formula that is determined by each state's statute.

- Temporary total disability payments replace wages lost while the injured worker is recovering. It varies by jurisdiction. Those on temporary total disability are unable to work initially, but are expected to fully recover.
- Permanent total disability payments replace future income lost by workers who are unable to work again because of industrial injury or occupation disease.
- Temporary partial disability is awarded to those who return to work on a restricted basis while awaiting maximum recovery.
- Permanent partial disability reflects the difference between income a worker could earn with a job-caused disability and previous income.

It is the intent of the system to effect a prompt return to work. In order to return to one's job, the injured employee must be able to (1) travel to and from work, (2) be at work for an amount of time expected by the employer and (3) perform the tasks and duties of a job for which the employer is willing to pay a full wage or salary. However, for many different reasons, some disabled or injured workers remain on disability for unusually long periods of time. Many never return to work. For those with a permanent medical impairment, workers' compensation systems generally provide for some indemnity benefit. For some, psychological factors often complicate a speedy return to work. Recovery from a physical injury requires more than physical healing. Depression, pain, anxiety, discouragement, distress may exacerbate or prolong the healing process. A psychological evaluation may help the injured workers and may also serve to uncover those who are manipulative or intent on defrauding the system.

Workers' Compensation and the Americans with Disabilities Act

The Americans with Disabilities Act of 1990 (ADA) was enacted with the intent to eliminate discrimination against individuals with disabilities or functional impairments. Title I of the ADA specifies that employers, employment agencies, labor organizations or joint labor-management committees may not discriminate against any qualified individual with a disability. Much of what was set out in the Rehabilitation Act of 1973 was incorporated in the ADA. In brief, the employer must make "reasonable accommodations" for the disabled. The effect of the ADA on workers' compensation is unclear at this time. Of potential contentious issue is the question of whether the employee can perform a certain job and, if not, what modifications could be made to allow the individual to return to work.

Extent of the Problem

Statistics compiled by the Bureau of Labor Statistics have shown a steady annual increase in workplace injuries and illnesses. Over 6.6 million injuries and illnesses were reported by the early 1990s. The National Safety Council's statistics on occupational injury and illness incidence per 100 full-time workers for *all* industries was 8.79 in 1990. Thirty-eight percent of all injuries were to the trunk of the body, 29.2% to the upper extremities, 21.7% to the lower extremities, 5.9% to the head and neck, and 5.2% to multiple body parts.

Who are these injured workers? One survey by Intracorp conducted in 1995 found that nearly 12% of all workers surveyed said that they had a work-related injury or illness during the past three years. Of this, 73% had lost time from work. Workers who suffered an on-the-job injury lost an average of 33 days from work while ill workers lost an average of 25 days. Table II shows that while 30% of those injured were out of work for less than one week, 25% were out of work for more than three months and 10% have never returned to work. Those workers with job-related injuries or illnesses were significantly more likely than the general employee in the workforce to work for smaller employers and to have worked a shorter period of time on the job (less than four years). Of those suffering from a work-related illness, most (33%) were off work for one to four weeks and 17% never returned to work. The most commonly cited injuries include back problems, broken bones, cuts and carpal tunnel syndrome. Ill workers, more likely to be female, suffer from stress and allergies.

Researchers from the National Bureau of Economic Research analyzed data from the Minnesota workers' compensation system and found that certain types of injuries were more likely to arise on Mondays than other weekdays, leading to the speculation that some employees who were injured over the weekend reported their injuries as having occurred at work. An alternative explanation is that after the weekend hiatus, workers are more prone to injure themselves. Findings also showed that employers were no more likely to deny liability for Monday injury claims than for those occurring on other weekdays. There appears to be more than meets the eye here, and the "Monday effect" may be just an anomaly.

TABLE II

Time Lost From Work for Work-Related Illness and Injury

LOST TIME	PERCENTAGE OF INJURED AND ILL WORKERS	
	INJURY	ILLNESS
<1 day	11%	6%
2-7 days	19	17
1-4 weeks	17	33
1-3 months	18	13
>3 months	25	14
Still out of work	10	17

Source: Intracorp, Berwyn, Pa., May 1995.

Spiraling Costs

To understand the nature and extent of the costs of workers' compensation, it helps to compare them to health care costs. During the 1980s, for example, national expenditures for health care rose by 117%, causing employers and insurers to scramble for cost-containment measures. During this same time period, and without public out-cry or corporate concern, health expenditures for workers' compensation rose 191%! Nothing was done; there were no calls for investigation or action.

In 1993, employers spent $70 billion on workers' compensation according to the National Council on Compensation Insurance. Workers' compensation has become one of the most onerous and uncontrollable costs associated with doing business in America. Typically, there is no dollar limit on the total amount of medical care for workers' compensation claimants and, as stated, workers' compensation laws forbid employers from charging a copayment or deductible for medical care reimbursements. Not surprisingly, then, employers are targeting disability and workers' compensation costs. And, workers' compensation is ripe for cost cutting.

It costs no more to provide health care to workers' compensation patients than to other patients, holding constant the extent of injury, use of service and personal characteristics of patients. The problem is a lack of price discrimination. Employers, employees and insurers do not usually scrutinize or challenge medical expenses; providers know that the cost of medical services will be unchallenged and, unfortunately, some charge more. Indeed, a study measuring the cost difference between workers' compensation and standard health insurance in Minnesota found that workers' compensation claimants incurred higher medical costs than did claimants for nonwork-related causes. Charges per service were also higher for workers' compensation claimants, in particular, X-ray charges.

Between 1985 and 1993, the average medical cost of a workers' compensation claim increased from $3,800 to $8,700. Costs are separated into medical and nonmedical (indemnity) expenses such as vocational rehabilitation, death benefits and the different types of disability cited above. In 1990, medical costs per case averaged $6,611 compared to $3,673 in 1985. Indemnity costs per case averaged $12,833 in 1990, an increase from $7,773 in 1985.

Part of the problem is that employees view workers' compensation as a right that is inviolate. But, with costs rising geometrically, action must be taken albeit without disturbing the sacred trust between employer and employee and without violating state law. States, for example, have started to crack down on job injury costs by tightening the eligibility rules for collecting disability benefits, limiting recourse to the courts, addressing fraud and, in some cases, cutting benefits. (See Table III.) Both Texas and California, states with very high workers' compensation claims, have shown dramatic improvement in containing workers' compensation costs. In California, for example, high rates were driven by the high frequency of claims in general and an excessive number of mental stress claims. Exorbitant litigation costs and fraud were also factors. Reform has resulted in an assault on fraud, controls on system abuses, and requirements that limit stress claims. These reforms have resulted in the reduction in net costs of workers' compensation in this state.

Organized labor, however, has argued that the pendulum has shifted too far in favor of the employers. Some severely injured workers were not receiving adequate compensation care. Clearly, cutting benefits is not the only nor necessarily the best way to reduce the costs of workers' compensation. There are more humane means of achieving similar results.

Return-to-Work Policies

Potential savings can be realized by returning an injured or sick worker to the job as quickly and as feasibly as possible. Disability payments to off-the-job workers account for 60% of total workers' compensation outlays. Many surveys have shown that the average injured or ill worker remains off the job three to four times longer than medically necessary. In the vast majority of these cases, recovery and return to work can occur within a few

TABLE III

State Experience With Reining in Workers' Compensation Costs

ARKANSAS
> **You can't be vague anymore:** Previously, all a worker had to do was describe an injury; now the exact time and place of the mishap are required.

> **You can't complain about pain anymore:** An aching back from too much lifting at work? Don't bother citing it in a claim if there is no underlying injury; the state no longer considers pain a factor in calculating a disability.

> **You can't blame your employer for the ravages of time anymore:** If a disability is caused or prolonged by a preexisting condition or the natural process of aging, benefits are reduced accordingly.

FLORIDA
> **You can't pay your lawyer as much anymore:** Injured workers must take complaints to an arbitrator first. After that, lawyers can take cases, but their fees have been reduced to 20% of the first $5,000 of benefits awarded, 15% of the next $5,000 and 10% of anything higher than that.

OREGON
> **You can't choose your doctor anymore:** Employers can establish mandatory managed care programs for injured workers.

CONNECTICUT
> **You can't plead mental anguish anymore:** The state will no longer award disability benefits for mental or psychological disorders unless they are accompanied by a physical injury.

> **You can't get relief from inflation anymore:** Cost-of-living adjustments have been eliminated from disability benefits.

CALIFORNIA
> **You can't get benefits for a hectic life anymore:** For a worker to claim a disability because of stress, the strains of the workplace must be the predominant cause. Previously job irritants counted if they contributed to just 10% of the stress.

TEXAS
> **You can't collect benefits as easily anymore:** To qualify for special supplemental benefits, a worker must be at least 15% disabled, based on an American Medical Association test gauging general physical condition, not ability to work. Few pass.

Source: New York Times, 3/16/95.

working days. Eight in ten injured workers who begin a rehabilitation program within four months of being injured successfully return to work. Savings from return-to-work programs can have a big payoff. Northwestern National Life Insurance Company found that for every $1 spent on rehabilitation, $96 was saved in disability payments.

Utilization of Cost-Efficient Providers

Under the present system, the injured employee has no incentive to choose a cost-efficient provider. Reimbursement for medical care is statutorily regulated and is still based on fee for service. Providers, constrained by managed care for non-workers' compensation patients, will charge higher fees to treat workers' compensation patients. Their use of medical technology is also greater in their treatment of workers' compensation cases.

Elimination of Fraud

It is not an isolated situation where the injured or ill worker can make more money by staying on disability than by returning to work. One large publishing company found that employees who were getting workers' compensation were receiving 115% of their salary! Double dipping must be eliminated. Employers should deduct workers' compensation from a duplication in company payments. If an employee is also receiving disability payments, he or she should not also be entitled to workers' compensation. In some states, employees receiving workers' compensation can qualify also for unemployment benefits. Employers should offer workers transitional jobs even with their physical restrictions.

Older workers who receive workers' compensation may retire during their convalescence. Some collect their pension *and* continue to receive workers' compensation. Employers must eliminate any disincentive to working such as occupational injury pay supplements.

Other aspects of fraud include the injured employee who is collecting benefits but is also working at another job, and the injured employee who is collecting benefits but is physically able to return to work.

Review of Short-Term Disability Coverage

Short-term disability (STD) claims do not receive the same scrutiny that medical, dental or long-term disability claims do. The former are probably the most abused benefits offered by employers. Claims review would help an employer understand the scope of overpayment and the type of problems resulting in an STD claim being filed.

Managed Workers' Compensation

Employer involvement in managing workers' compensation can yield significant cost savings. As managed care has transformed the way health care is delivered and financed, it has generally ignored the workers' compensation industry. Part of the reason is the significant differences in the two industries. However, many are now realizing that managed care principles can be applied to workers' compensation. The following strategies can be implemented, although in some cases changes in state laws may be necessary:

- Utilize providers who are cost-efficient. Many managed workers' compensation firms offer the injured worker a choice of providers who have signed agreements with them. This concept has been the basis of managed care.

- Establish medical fee schedules to restrict physician reimbursement in an effort to stem the cost shifting.
- Establish a hospital fee schedule.
- Conduct bill audits to detect unauthorized charges.
- Rely on a case manager to coordinate the process. The case manager is the liaison between the injured worker and the medical provider. Coordinating care is an excellent means of monitoring the care rendered, the costs of such care and the injured worker's progress.
- Establish a fraud detection program.
- Require a second opinion after three months if the injured employee is still collecting workers' compensation.

Sensing a void, managed care entities are attacking the workers' compensation market with a vengeance. Indeed, the involvement of managed care organizations in workers' compensation increased dramatically from 1994 to 1995, and HMOs are becoming more adept at providing services such as loss prevention and third party administration. Employers should be very careful in selecting a managed workers' compensation organization because many lack experience with workers' compensation or cannot handle the administrative requirements internally. The cost structure, too, is quite different from straight health insurance. The field is still too young to make assessments or pronouncements; however, the next few years should be interesting to see how this new concept evolves.

Twenty-Four Hour Coverage

Other ideas designed to address the problems inherent in the system include 24-hour coverage. Under this scheme, individuals would be covered by one health insurance plan around the clock, regardless of the origin of the impairment. The typical 24-hour coverage plan would roll the medical component of workers' compensation into traditional employer-provided health insurance for off-work injuries. Most 24-hour coverage plans also permit employers to use coinsurance and deductibles for work-related injuries. The indemnity portion of workers' compensation would not change. To date, 24-hour coverage has not been implemented in any state, suggesting that substantial administrative and/or political barriers exist. One major barrier is the Employee Retirement Income Security Act (ERISA), which preempts states from regulating employee benefit plans but grants exemptions solely for the purpose of meeting state workers' compensation statutes. The full impact of ERISA on 24-hour coverage has never been tested in the courts, and the possibility of problems may frighten potential proponents and slow down the work of those attempting to move forward with this idea.

What Can the Employer Do?

One should not be a passive player in this area. The stakes are too high, both financially and in human terms. It is widely believed that an active concern for employee health and well-being generally leads to a decrease in rates of disability claims. Low-loss organizations are characterized by their strong commitment to safety and accident prevention. The organization's systematic monitoring and correcting of unsafe behavior, their use of safety training, and their programs to help the injured worker return to work all contribute to low accident rates. Those organizations with no meaningful safety and health programs, those with poor communication networks and no viable safety training programs are generally characterized as high-loss organizations.

Several easy steps can and should be taken to rein in the costs of workers' compensation.

1. Be sure that the injured or ill employee receives immediate medical assistance. Delays can prolong recovery and increase costs.
2. Report the incident quickly to the insurance carrier. A study by ITT Hartford found that medical care and lost wage payments cost one-third less on average when an injury or illness is reported shortly after it happens.
3. Intervene early and maintain contact with the injured employee while he or she is recuperating. Many injured employees are out longer than necessary because no one encourages them to return to work.
4. Make light duty or substitute employment available, if possible.
5. Learn from the injury/accident. What can be changed to avoid recurrence?
6. Reduce the incentives for a lawsuit. Lawsuits prolong the claim settlement, delay the worker's return to work and increase costs. Conflict resolution may avoid a protracted, costly legal battle.

But, the best way to reduce the cost of your workers' compensation costs is to prevent employees from being hurt on the job in the first place. Safety should be the employer's number one concern.

CHAPTER 9

Retiree Benefits: Who Will Take Care of Me When I'm Old?

In the late 1980s, this author wrote a book entitled *Retiree Health Care: A Ticking Time Bomb.* Since that time, we have all gotten older and the issue of retiree health benefits has become more complex and contentious. The time bomb is still ticking away. As health expenditures increase, and as the number of retirees grows, serious problems such as how to finance this benefit and how to meet the needs of retirees beg for attention and resolution.

Employer-sponsored retiree health plans were never intended to be the primary source of retirement health insurance. Rather, they were designed to supplement Medicare benefits. Basically, these plans provide coverage for retirees who are not yet eligible for Medicare or supplement Medicare benefits for those age 65 and older. These benefits are part of the earned compensation of current and future retirees. Over time, these programs have grown from relative obscurity to a significant feature in the benefits package of most employers. But, uncertainties in estimating the cost of postretirement medical plans complicate projecting future retiree health care costs. The major difficulties stem from cost fluctuations due to changes in price levels for specific services, cost changes resulting from developments in medical technology and cost changes resulting from changes in Medicare benefits and/or reimbursement procedures. For the most part, it is the employer that is at risk for the majority of the costs.

The amount spent on retiree benefits is significant and is increasing substantially each year. For many employers, health care costs are greater than pension costs. As the baby boom generation approaches retirement age, the potential costs of retiree benefits are staggering: Estimates of unfunded liability associated with employer-sponsored retiree health benefits suggest that future unfunded liabilities could total over $2 trillion.

Most medium sized and large companies provide health insurance to their retirees; but, employers are very concerned about current costs and the implied future liability of those promised benefits. How to control the costs of retiree health benefits, how to fund for future retiree medical benefits, how to predict actuarially an organization's obligation to its retirees, and the legal issues of protecting workers from losing a benefit (the disenfranchised employee) are major issues that merit an employer's attention.

Employees, too, are worried. In particular, the possibility of employers eliminating or reducing promised benefits have left many retirees, and those close to retirement, very concerned. Since Medicare does not cover all costs, a retiree health package is very important. Private coverage is prohibitively expensive for most and, for those with a preexisting condition, affordable insurance is usually impossible to obtain. Hence, for retirees and their dependents, regardless of their age, having medical coverage provides retirement security against expensive medical costs.

This chapter will explore the costs of providing retiree health benefits, the legal implications of changing one's retiree health plan, the implications of managed Medicare, and how all these factors affect employers and retirees alike. While the issue is multifaceted and complex, unwillingness to confront the situation could have extremely serious financial consequences for employers and retirees.

Demographic Considerations

The implications of the aging population on financing retiree health care benefits are tremendous. Knowledge of basic demographics clearly illustrates the seriousness of the situation. In 1980, there were 26 million Americans over the age of 65; in 1995, there were 33 million; and by 2020, it is estimated that there will be 52 million individuals over age 65. The aging of the population will clearly have a dramatic effect on the health care and social service systems. In particular, the "oldest old," those 85 years and older, is the fastest growing cohort. The number of those age 85 and older is expected to more than double within the next decade!

The demographic structure of the population has made this issue a ticking time bomb. As the baby boom generation ages, a significant number of employees will reach retirement age at the same time. The ratio of elderly persons to persons of working age is also a serious consideration because individuals are living longer and families are having fewer children. The situation changes the shape of the elderly support ratio (the dependency ratio, which is the number of those 65 and older compared to those 18-64 years). The specter of funding retiree benefits to an ever-increasing pool of retirees is staggering. The average male worker reaching age 65 in the year 2030, for example, will require an additional 25 monthly payments of any promised benefit compared to a male age 65 retiring in 1990. The average female worker reaching age 65 in 2030 will require an additional 39 monthly payments.

Characteristics of Retiree Health Plans

Employer-sponsored health plans are recognized by ERISA as welfare benefits and are part of the national fabric of health insurance. As the probability of incurring medical expenses increases with age, the value of this insurance relative to the fixed income and assets of most retirees also increases. Not surprisingly, there is wide variation among employer-sponsored retiree health plans. Most offer hospital and medical benefits that generally are considered to be Medicare wraparound plans (coverage designed to supplement Medicare payments) for those age 65 and older. For retirees under age 65, coverage is often identical to that of active employees. In almost all plans, coverage tends to follow the acute care orientation of the Medicare program, and long-term care needs beyond limited skilled nursing home health services after hospitalization are not covered.

In virtually all cases, the benefit is structured as a defined benefit, which means that payments are determined by actual service use rather than by specified dollar amounts. Lifetime dollar limits or maximum annual out-of-pocket expenses might be specified in some plans. For those 65 and older, employer-sponsored retiree health plans can be one of three types: (1) coordination-of-benefits plans, (2) supplement plans and (3) carve-out plans. Coordination-of-benefits plans pay the difference between what Medicare pays and the actual cost of services, up to what the plan would pay without Medicare. Under a Medicare supplement plan, payment is made for defined services not covered by Medicare. The plan may impose coinsurance and deductibles. Under a carve-out plan, payment equals what the employer's plan would pay for those under age 65 minus the Medicare benefit. Carve-out plans may also require the same copayments and deductibles from retirees as from active employees. Carve-out plans are the most common, and it is widely held that they result in the lowest plan costs but the highest beneficiary cost of the three plan types.

Eligibility for retiree health plan coverage varies with age and length of service. In general, those who have worked in larger firms, those covered by collective bargaining agreements and those with higher levels of pre-retirement income have a far greater likelihood of benefiting from employer-sponsored health benefits. Entitlement is predicated on actual retirement from the organization or disability retirement. Employees who do not meet the requirements for benefits at retirement or who leave the organization before they retire usually do not qualify for health benefits. Coverage of spouses and dependents of current and deceased retirees also varies by company. Employers are most likely to cover dependents if the plans are contributory for these beneficiaries. The benefit, at the moment, is not portable, which means employees who leave cannot credit their time with another employer.

Cost Factors

Most employers pay retiree health costs as part of their operating costs as opposed to establishing a fund for this purpose. Not surprisingly, payment for coverage varies. Some employers subsidize the full cost of the premium while others require a deductible and/or payment from their retirees and/or dependents. However, in response to the huge increases in health insurance costs, many employers have sought to implement cost sharing by increasing the employees' share of premiums and deductibles.

A Foster and Higgins survey found that the 1993 medical plan cost for all retirees averaged $2,755 per retiree. Of those employers that separated costs for retirees by age category, the costs for those under age 65 totaled $5,216 versus $1,786 for retirees 65 years and older. Since Medicare is the primary payer of benefits for retirees age 65 and older, it is logical that the employer's costs would be less. However, the Medicare integration method, which determines how the retiree and employer split the remaining expenses after Medicare benefits are paid, can and does have a significant impact on employer liability.

Recently issued financial standards have highlighted the mounting obligations associated with this benefit; many employers have had to reconsider their policy in this area. Most employers have made one or more changes in the past few years to control retirees health care costs: increasing retiree contributions in the form of copayments and/or deductibles, requiring managed care, reducing the lifetime benefit cap and capping the employer contribution. A small percentage canceled the benefits altogether for future retirees or for those who had retired after a specified date. Indeed, statistics show that there has been a gradual erosion in the number of employers offering retiree coverage over time. Between 1988 and 1994, for example, the proportion of retirees with health coverage declined from 44% to 34%. The decline is a result of an overall decline in employer-sponsored retiree health benefits.

As a general rule, the larger the corporation the more likely that retiree benefits will be offered; however, as of 1995 fewer than half of large employers offer health coverage to retirees. Small employers are much less likely to offer such coverage and, of those who do, the retirees are much more likely to pay the full cost of their coverage than those who worked for large employers.

Large employers generally use a carve-out, under which Medicare's payment is subtracted from the employer plan's normal benefit or from the total expense before normal benefits are calculated. Small employers generally use coordination of benefits, under which Medicare is treated as a separate plan and a claimant may receive up to 100% of expenses through a combination of Medicare benefits and employer plan benefits.

As Congress debates Medicare reform, employers are worried that changes could translate into additional costs for them. For example, an increase in the Part B deductible would directly increase costs for employers whose retiree health plans are coordinated with Medicare. If Congress passes a Medicare reduction spending bill, providers would shift almost $92 billion in payment reductions to private payers in terms of higher private insurance premiums. The National Leadership Coalition on Health Care estimated that employer health spending would increase by $75 billion from 1996 through 2002, and employee contributions for employer health coverage would increase by $6.4 billion over the same period due to cost shifting.

The coalition estimated that $66 billion of the $75 billion increase in employer costs due to cost shifting would be passed on to workers in the form of lost wage growth and equal approximately $1,000 per covered worker over the six-year time period. It is logical that coverage would decline among firms that see an increase in premiums as a result of this increased cost shifting. The coalition further estimated that .5 million people would lose insurance coverage due to increased cost shifting, which includes over half of this figure whose employers would discontinue coverage, a chilling prospect.

Another troubling issue is the prospect of sharply increasing the annual Medicare portion of payroll taxes that would be required to keep the

Medicare Hospital Insurance Trust Fund solvent. On a more positive note, however, potential savings to employers could be the option of retirees receiving coverage through managed care plans with the federal government directly paying the beneficiary's premium to the managed care organization. These retirees, theoretically, would have little interest in or need of employer-provider health plans that supplement Medicare. A discussion of Medicare managed care is forthcoming.

Cost Liability Issues

Employers tend to view retiree health benefits from a perspective of how to manage these rapidly rising costs. The lack of funding for this benefit is considered to be more of a financial problem than pension funding was in the early 1970s. Part of the problem is the difficulty in actuarially calculating future health care costs. Evidence suggests that almost none of the retiree health benefits promised to current and future retirees is funded. Without funding and benefit guarantees, retirees are still at risk to lose all or part of the promised benefit. Without passing judgment on the lack of foresight of most employers in this area, the fact remains that many neither anticipated nor planned for the rising liability they now face and are largely unprepared to fund the promised benefit.

Compounding the problem is the fact that individuals are retiring earlier and living longer in their retirement years. It was not that long ago when workers generally retired at age 65 and usually died a few years thereafter. Now individuals are retiring earlier and living well into their 80s. A 1991 Northwestern National Life Insurance Company study found that cutbacks in companies' retirement health benefits could expose many future retirees to bankruptcy. Looking at average out-of-pocket annual expenses after retirement, many will see their nest egg depleted before they reach age 80.

The greatest threat to economic security is the high out-of-pocket cost of medical care, and older individuals are the heaviest users of health services. Living on fixed and relatively lower income, many find it difficult to budget for uncertain future health expenditures. Many are unprepared financially and emotionally for the potential costs of medical expenses in retirement years. Compounding their worries is the nagging question of whether their retiree benefits will be there when needed. Clearly the economic climate should provide the impetus for employers to focus attention on their ability to meet its obligations.

Accounting Considerations

Much of the controversy and uncertainty surrounding the provision of health benefits to retirees stems from recent changes in accounting standards and tax laws. Both of these factors exert enormous influence on everyday business practices: Accounting standards shape an organization's financial profile and expected profitability. Any requirement that increases liabilities is clearly unwelcome.

The Financial Accounting Standards Board (FASB)—the entity that sets standards that define current accounting practice—ruled that employers must recognize and disclose the unfunded liability for future post-employment health benefits in their annual financial reports. FAS 106 had sent shivers through corporate boardrooms. FAS 106 requires companies to calculate retiree nonpension benefit costs on an accrual basis rather than the previously common pay-as-you-go basis. By 1993, 97% of Fortune 500 companies studied by Buck Consultants had already adopted FAS 106 and, of this percentage, 73% elected immediate recognition of the transition obligation. Twenty-three percent of the companies that have already adopted FAS 106 have plan assets; two-thirds of these companies have funded only 20% or less of their postretirement nonpension benefit liability. A 1995 survey of FAS 106 results shows little rise in retiree health care expensed in 1994.

Evidence indicates that recognizing obligations for past service liabilities on the balance sheet resulted in write-downs of 7-12% in book value among Standard & Poor's 500 companies alone. Also, the accrued liabilities, most of which are unfunded, will ultimately have to be paid, even though the impact on financial statements has been noncash accounting charges. It appears that many companies are using lower medical cost trend rates and lower discount rates in reporting their financial liability for postretirement benefits as required by FAS 106. Discount rates dropped from 1992 to 1993 from an average 8.14% to 7.31%. Of greater impact was the decline in the medical cost trend rate, reflecting the general drop in annual health cost increases.

FAS 112, also adopted by FASB, requires that companies accrue the cost and recognize the liability for providing benefits to former or inactive employees after employment but before retirement. Less than one-third of the companies studied by Buck Consultants have adopted FAS 112; three-quarters of the companies that have not yet adopted FAS 112 did not expect it to have any material impact.

In summary, while accounting standards now require employers to disclose their liability for retiree health benefits, many employers have questioned, or are now questioning, both their original commitment to providing this benefit and their ability to prefund. Legally, however, an employer must beware of the pitfalls of reneging on its obligation. The consequences could be serious.

Legal Considerations

Since the 1950s, many companies have provided health insurance coverage to retirees even though there was no legal obligation to do so. The high cost of postretirement health care (relative to the modest incomes of most retirees) provided the impetus for the establishment of retiree health insurance benefits. Employers and employees alike considered the benefit as a quid pro quo for continuous, dedicated service. Post-Medicare, employers continued to offer coverage as a supplement to Medicare. At the time, the cost was relatively inexpensive. The climate began to change in the 1970s and 1980s.

The tenuousness of retiree health benefits was vividly demonstrated in 1986. The LTV Corporation, at the time the nation's second largest steel producer, filed for reorganization under Chapter 11 of the U.S. Bankruptcy Code. Desperately short of cash after losing more than $1.5 billion in five years, LTV chose bankruptcy because it saw no prospect for a fast turnaround in the domestic steel industry's extended slump. In an effort to cut expenses, LTV's immediate plan was to terminate health and life insurance benefits to more than 78,000 of its retirees. This action propelled Congress to secure these benefits by enacting a series of bills to protect not only LTV's retirees, but also others in potentially similar situations.

The intent of congressional action was to ensure the continuation of health coverage for retiring or retired employees. Additionally, Congress intended to ensure that the bankruptcy court permit the use of income resulting from tax credits to pay for health and life benefits for retirees. The LTV case highlighted what could happen when an employer declares bankruptcy or suddenly chooses to terminate its health plan for retirees. After the LTV crisis, there were other court challenges filed by other employers. Rulings tended to be specifically related to the unique facts in each case and, as such, have served to raise serious questions about employers' obligations and responsibilities regarding retiree health benefits. In the majority of decisions, the courts have concluded that retiree health benefits were intended to be vested at retirement unless the company made it clear that it did not intend to provide lifetime coverage or clearly reserved its right to terminate or amend benefits.

More recently, when John Morrill and Co., a meat packing company, announced that it was ending health insurance coverage for its 3,300 retirees and their families, the United Food and Commercial Workers (UFCW) union filed suit. The Morrill workers contended that they were promised health coverage for life and that the company's actions were in violation of this agreement. The Eighth Circuit Court of Appeals ruled that the promise of lifetime health benefits expires every time a labor contract is renewed *unless* the contract language is specific *even if* the company told retiring workers that they had lifetime benefits. The court viewed the expiration of a contract as the expiration of lifetime health insurance benefits unless the contract said otherwise. The UFCW, angered by the verdict, appealed the decision but the U.S. Supreme Court announced that it would not review the decision. Hence, the Eighth Circuit's decision is upheld.

Ironically, the same appeals court came to the opposite conclusion in a similar case against Dubuque Packing Co. only ten years ago. In this case, the court ruled that Dubuque Packing was obligated to pay lifetime benefits to its retirees. Until the law is clarified, each employer should review carefully its contract language *before* terminating benefits.

There are no simple solutions to this complex issue. Given its emotional nature, the economic ramifications of termination to the retiree and the financial consequences of an employer providing retiree benefits, it is evident that there is a need for judicial clarification to promote the security, continuity and accessibility of retiree health benefits to retirees as well as to protect the financial health of the employer. What is clear, however, is that employers that generally believed that they had great flexibility and control over terminating health benefits for retirees had better think again. Employers must be aware of benefit plan document language regarding the provision of retiree medical benefits; court challenges most certainly will be waged and both employer and retiree should consult legal counsel.

Medicare Managed Care—Is It the Answer?

Maneuvering among legal, accounting and cost constraints is difficult at best. Managed Medicare plans have been touted as a possible solution to the problem. The concept is not new per se, but only recently has interest been shown.

Congress created the Medicare risk contract program in 1982 to try to capitalize on the potential cost savings with HMOs. As designed, HMOs would be paid a flat fee for each Medicare beneficiary enrolled, the law setting HMO payments for comprehensive care at 95% of the estimated average cost to Medicare of treating the patients in the fee-for-service sector. For over a decade, this rate setting system has been used even though the flaws were well-known. Specifically, because HMO payment rates are fixed, Medicare cannot lower rates through competition or share in any savings that HMOs achieve through greater efficiency. Also, HMO payment rates are not adequately risk adjusted to reflect cost differences deriving from differences in health status. Consequently, Medicare has paid HMOs more than it would have for the same patients' care under fee for service! HMOs that can attract Medicare enrollees and provide health care for less than the capitated rate keep the difference. As such, Medicare risk contracts are viewed as potentially lucrative and most managed care plans have launched an all-out war to enroll healthy Medicare beneficiaries for obvious reasons. Managed care's profits are maximized, indeed assured, under the present system.

Despite serious negative factors (no competitive bidding, no negotiating with HMOs over rates, inability to modify the rates), there has been a steady pattern of growth in the number of plans contracting with the Health Care Financing Administration (no surprise since a Medicare contract is lucrative) as well as the number of individuals enrolling in Medicare managed care plans. As of January 1, 1995, over 3 million beneficiaries, or 9% of the total Medicare population, were enrolled in a managed care plan. By region, more than half of Medicare beneficiaries enrolled in such plans reside in California, Arizona, Nevada and Hawaii. More recently, there has been an increase in growth in Florida and other southern states. In the state of Florida alone, in less than one year (1994), HMO enrollment increased from 2.4 million to 2.8 million. Thirteen percent of the Medicare-eligible Floridians are in managed care, compared with the national average of 7%. Florida has been described by managed care operators as a "dream world for managed care."

What are the cost implications? A 1995 study by the Group Health Association of America and Price Waterhouse found that as the percentage of beneficiaries getting health care through the Medicare risk contract program grew, per capita costs for the Medicare fee-for-service program declined. They conclude that Medicare budgetary savings would be substantial if the Medicare risk program were to grow considerably. Other studies show that more could be done to maximize savings.

What does all this mean to the employer? A Towers Perrin survey of 30,000 retirees whose employers had switched from fee-for-service Medicare programs to managed care found that per capita cost savings averaged between $600 to $1,000. As more studies are undertaken, it will become clearer how cost-effective managed Medicare programs are. Actual experience in the program provides the best basis for assessing managed care's potential to effectively serve this population. At this writing, more needs to be documented regarding quality of care rendered, referral patterns (Are individuals being denied referrals to specialists or admittance to the hospital?) and patient satisfaction.

By far the most significant obstacle toward wider acceptance of the managed care option is the perceived lack of choice of doctor and the perceived idea that managed care provides inferior care. If this concept is to succeed in the long term, there must be more education and information about the program. Discussion about available plans, payment policies, choice and access must be made available. Relatively few Medicare beneficiaries and pre-Medicare beneficiaries are aware of how managed care functions under Medicare. Most, for example, are not aware that Medicare risk members are permitted to leave the program at any time.

An American Health Services Research book, *HMOs and the Elderly*, published in 1994, is a good guidebook. The book focuses on costs and use of services, enrollee satisfaction, quality of care for specific conditions, appropriate premium levels and Medicare risk contracting. Another guidebook published by Aspen Publishing, *Essentials of Managed Health Care*, is an excellent introduction to the concepts of managed care and discusses the unique requirements of Medicare among other topics.

Retirees' Need for Long-Term Care

Without detracting from the severity of the problem of managing the costs of retiree health benefits, it is important to mention the equally large problem of long-term care (LTC). As longevity is increasing, so too is the likelihood of developing diseases and conditions of old age such as Alzheimer's and other dementias; arthritis; Parkinson's; stroke; and chronic illnesses such as diabetes, chronic obstructive lung disease, hypertension, and ischemic heart disease. Each does not necessarily shorten life, but certainly takes a toll on the ability to live an independent one. It is estimated that more than half of those 65 years and older will eventually need some form of extended care. Stated more dramatically, by 2020, the Health Insurance Association of America says that more than 12 million elderly Americans will need some sort of long-term care.

No single factor sparks the demand for long-term care. Rather, a number of factors, each associated with a specific aspect of a chronic illness, produces the demand. But, when a chronic illness strikes, most older Americans find the long-term care services they need are not covered by Medicare, other public programs or private Medigap insurance.

Medicare actually accounts for only a small portion of the nation's expenditures for nursing home care; primarily it provides acute care coverage for those age 65 and older, particularly hospital and surgical care and accompanying periods of recovery. Table I illustrates the percent distribution of Medicare payments by type of service. The numbers clearly show a decrease in the proportion of payments for inpatient hospitalization and skilled nursing care, but a huge increase in payments for home health care and outpatient services. Yet, most elderly believe that Medicare's coverage in-

TABLE I

Percent Distribution of Medicare Program Payments by Type of Service: 1967 and 1993

	1967	1993
Inpatient Hospital	62.1%	52.7%
Skilled Nursing Care	6.5	3.3
Home Health Agency	1.0	7.5
Physician	28.9	26.9
Outpatient	0.9	9.6

Source: HCFA, data from the Medical Decision Support System.

cludes basic LTC services. Because of this erroneous belief, most do not feel that they have to save for their health care needs once they reach age 65.

One does not have to be an economist to realize the gravity of the situation. Those with $1 million in liquid assets can get away without any type of long-term coverage because they can pay for it as needed. Those with a more modest net worth will exhaust their resources fairly quickly. Presently, many elderly and/or their families pay out of pocket, making long-term care services the single largest threat to their financial security. For example, a year of nursing home care at private pay rates costs approximately $80,000, a figure which exceeds the assets (excluding principal residence) of more than half of the elderly. Less than half of elderly persons admitted to nursing homes are able to enter as private payers and remain in that category. One-quarter are eligible for Medicaid at admission and 14% eventually "spend down" their assets to qualify for Medicaid benefits.

A study conducted by researchers at the Agency for Health Care Policy Research estimated that 6% of all individuals who turn 65 years of age in 1995 will enter nursing homes and spend down while there. About three times as many women as men will spend down to Medicaid in nursing homes, and twice as many women will be Medicaid recipients by final discharge.

Since Medicare does not fully cover all medical costs, most older Americans purchase supplemental medical insurance, or Medigap policies. More than two-thirds of the 37 million Americans covered by Medicare have Medigap insurance. This supplemental coverage is often provided on a group basis—mainly through retirees' former employers or the American Association of Retired Persons. These policies are typically designed to supplement Medicare's coverage of acute care costs, not LTC costs. Indeed, the extent of the LTC coverage provided by such policies has been limited. There are ten standard Medigap policies, covering items such as prescription drugs, skilled nursing care and the 20% of doctor bills not covered by Medicare.

Reflecting increases in health care costs, the Medigap premiums have also increased. Much of the rise in premiums is attributed to increased use of outpatient services (Medicare pays the full cost of much in-hospital care, but beneficiaries pay at least 20% of the cost of outpatient services). Average premiums range from $51 to $152 per month, depending on how much the policies cover. Rate increases may encourage more Medicare beneficiaries to enroll in HMOs, which accept Medicare fees as payment in full. But it may turn out that the sicker and older people will not be those who switch, thus providing the impetus for Medigap rates to rise even faster.

Ideally, LTC insurance should cover most nursing home care and/or home health care, including skilled nursing care at licensed skilled or intermediate care facilities, as well as intermediate care. Annual premiums for such policies depend on the scope of coverage and age at enrollment and are modeled along the lines of whole life insurance policies. There is no standard in policy costs and benefits at this time. Most policies will pay if an individual cannot perform two of five activities of daily living without help: i.e., bathing, dressing, eating, moving around, going to the bathroom.

Some employers have explored assisting employees to purchase such insurance prior to retirement. But, despite the noteworthy developments in this area, there are still significant barriers to the widespread adoption of LTC insurance including price, administrative costs, fear of employee pressure for employer plan contribution and fear of government mandates for employer contributions to the plan.

Long-term care services involve both medical and nonmedical services, including rehabilitative, medical and supportive social services of various kinds for those who have functional limitations or chronic health conditions who need ongoing health care or assistance with normal activities of daily living. Such services include nursing home care and a range of home and community-based services: for example, visiting nurse, homemaker and delivered meals services, or adult day care.

LTC services incorporate the needs of two different types of individuals: those who have been discharged from a hospital and those with chronic conditions requiring care for an extended period of time. In fact, nursing home care absorbs over 77% of total LTC spending. Trends in utilization of skilled nursing facilities show that from 1972 through 1988, Medicare skilled nursing facilities (SNF) accounted for only 1-2% of all Medicare payments. Since that time, SNF payments soared from $1.8 billion to $4.4 billion in

1993. Why? The passage of the Medicare Catastrophic Coverage Act of 1988 marked the most significant expansion of the Medicare program.

This act was a catalyst that changed the SNF care environment by bringing more SNFs and beds into the Medicare program. Also, earlier legislation (the Omnibus Budget Reconciliation Act of 1987—OBRA) resulted in a standardized criteria for all nursing homes participating in federal programs, which changed nursing and social work staffing standards leading to an increase in professional staff personnel. OBRA also led to an increase in the use of rehabilitation and nursing services in order to comply with the act's regulations. In sum, most of the redistribution of Medicare SNF covered charges (and the increase in the number of SNF admissions) is a result of these pieces of legislation.

In summary, neither significant public nor private improvements in LTC financing and delivery are imminent. In fact, total LTC expenditures and the amount that federal taxpayers fund under current law are projected to rise rapidly as a result of the aging of the baby boom generation, increase in life expectancy and rates of price increases for LTC services that exceed general inflation.

Current arrangements for financing and delivering LTC services include Medicaid, Medicare, the health care program of the Department of Veterans Affairs and private financing. Problems associated with this arrangement have led to a continuing debate about how to restructure LTC policy. Various proposals have been developed to address these issues, for the most part focusing on expanding financial protection against LTC costs. The debate will undoubtedly intensify, fueled by projected sharp increases in spending (public and private) for LTC services, but such a discussion is beyond the scope of this chapter and this book. Suffice it to say that no consensus has emerged on what the future structure should be or on the appropriate role of the government or the employer within that structure.

Cost-Containment Strategies

Two cost-containment measures have been promoted as means of addressing the LTC problem: managed care/case management and home health care. The former seeks to structure health care financing and delivery so that only necessary and appropriate care is provided. The objective is to reduce costs and to enhance the quality of care. Case management is already being applied in LTC in the form of ongoing assessment, prior authorization of services, and care coordination. For example, case management organizations usually try to substitute lower cost for higher cost home and community-based services, to negotiate prices, and to create improved incentives for assuring quality through the knowledge of client outcomes that ongoing assessments make available.

The savings per case have been impressive. Most recently, the role of case management has expanded to include patient therapy and outcome. A good case management program should include activities ranging from pre-admission to services rendered after hospitalization. Early warning systems and concurrent reviews are needed to cope with the high costs of illness and out-of-plan benefit alternatives. However, the goal should be to coordinate health care services on behalf of the patient, not merely to obtain lower cost services. Quality must be ensured.

Another approach to cost containment, home health care, has assumed renewed interest. Ironically, in years past, people were tended to at home; hospitals were where the very sick went to die. With technological advances making it more viable to treat the infirm at home, a huge new industry has emerged. Intravenous administration of nutrients, antibiotics and other medications can easily and safely be done at home. Today, more than 1,000 diagnoses can be treated by means of home infusion therapy.

Home health care is the fastest growing segment of a fast growing health care system. Since 1985, the number receiving such care courtesy of Medicare, the main payer for this service, has doubled from 1.6 million to 3.5 million. As the caseload has mushroomed, however, there is growing concern that home health care has gone beyond its original mission of re-habilitating hospital patients to now include those with chronic illnesses who need care for months and years. To qualify for Medicare home health care, an individual must be homebound and require skilled nursing care not just custodial services. The individual must also require only intermittent visits, not constant surveillance.

Home care services are often dictated by how severely an individual is impaired in ability to function, as well as by how able friends and family are to provide care. At a point where the burden to the family exceeds the family's emotional or physical resources, formal help is usually sought.

Not surprisingly, by the mid-1990s, the biggest single out-of-pocket expense is home care, which also happens to be one of the fastest growing components of Medicare expenditures. Average annual out-of-pocket spending among those 65 and older totaled $2,800. In 1988, Medicare payments for home health care benefits totaled $1.9 billion. By 1993, the total soared to $9.7 billion, a 400% increase. Concomitantly, there has been a significant rise in the number of Medicare home health care agency visits and payments per person. But, charges per visit increased less rapidly and did not contribute significantly to the rise in program expenditures.

Significant savings to the Medicare program are evident. By facilitat-

TABLE II

Hospital Versus Home Care—Cost per Month

Service	Cost of Hospital Care	Cost of Home Care	Savings
AIDS Care	$23,190	$2,820	$20,370
Cancer Chemotherapy	10,500	3,500	7,000
Chronic Obstructive Pulmonary Disease	3,600	600	3,000
Routine Skilled Nursing	2,000	750	1,250
Ventilator-Dependent Care	2,320	1,766	544

ing discharges from acute care and other institutional facilities, federal savings have been identified to be between $300-$2,300 per patient episode, according to a Lewin ICF 1991 study. Table II shows the cost per month for hospital care versus home care and the resultant savings. Intuitively, home health care has the potential for significant savings, but there are also potentials for cost over-runs.

Efforts are underway to address cost-containment strategies, which include institution of copayments; fraud and abuse detection, especially for unnecessary services including visits that were never made; and excessive spending for specific services such as providing oxygen for patients with breathing problems. A 1994 report issued by the Senate Committee on Aging estimated that 10% of all health charges were fraudulent. Medicare, which spent $14.5 billion on home care in 1995, could have lost $1.5 billion to fraud alone!

Home health care is expected to continue to rise substantially in the coming years. Patients favor recuperating at home, which tends to speed recovery. What is important to monitor, however, is quality: quality in terms of meeting the medical needs of the patient as well as the emotional needs. It is important to know how the home care is monitored, who is delivering the services, if they are credentialed and how reputable the provider is. For example, it is less expensive to provide health aide care rather than nursing care. For some patients, aides can easily tend to the physical and emotional needs; but, for others, those who are sicker, nursing care should be provided.

Summary

The issue of retiree health benefits, a growing problem in and of itself, must be considered in the context of the overall economic climate of the late

1980s and 1990s. A decade and more of spending, unprecedented borrowing and budget deficits has created a serious situation. The surge in health care costs, the rising number of retired individuals and the cutbacks in Medicare have focused attention on the issue. Additionally, huge unfunded liabilities for this benefit is a cause for concern. Legal challenges have not served to clarify the issue; instead, conflicting court rulings have served to muddle the situation.

Of key concern to retirees, present and future, is whether they will be able to receive the promised benefits during their retirement years. Medicare does not by itself meet all the financial needs of the elderly. In fact, as Medicare continues to shift costs to the beneficiary and as health care costs rise, retirees can expect to pay a greater proportion of their income for medical expenses.

Of key concern to employers is the vast sum of money that will be needed to provide retiree health benefits; the amount spent on this benefit is not insignificant and is increasing dramatically each year. Perhaps managed Medicare will provide an acceptable means of providing coverage. It is still too early in the game to make an intelligent assessment.

What is clear, however, is that there are no simple solutions to this complex issue. With Medicare threatened with insolvency in 2002, the urgency for resolution cannot be overemphasized. Indeed, it is a critical time to focus on the retiree of the future. What would help is a legislative and tax policy that would promote the security, continuity and accessibility of retiree health benefits concomitant with strong cost-management strategies.

CHAPTER 10

Evaluate and Communicate

As the delivery of health care gets more complicated, it is imperative that employers and employees have the information they need to make intelligent decisions. Managed care, if it is to work effectively, relies on an informed consumer. The majority of Americans report that they need a lot more information to help them select a specific health plan and a primary care physician. Surveys have shown that the majority of individuals say they do not have a good understanding of managed care and do not fully understand how to select a doctor from a managed care list. Employers, too, need information. Selection among competing health plans should be based on an interpretation of data; and, once a plan is chosen, employers should demand an assurance of continuous monitoring to assess how well the plan is working.

As the preceding chapters highlighted, it is now evident that managed care organizations, hospitals and other providers of care must demonstrate their ability not only to contain costs and utilization, but also to ensure high quality (as measured by outcomes research). In order to satisfy the demands of the payers of care, there has been a rush to quantify performance outcomes, patient satisfaction and cost savings. The flood of data can often be confusing and conflicting.

This chapter focuses on the need for evaluation as well as the need for educating employees about changes in the health plan. Communication is quite important in order for the benefit plan to be utilized effectively, and for satisfaction and compliance to remain high.

Need for Evaluation

Evaluation is a means by which a plan is examined and a judgment made about its effectiveness. Assessment of health care can monitor the delivery of high-quality care as well as provide a tool for controlling costs. Since each organization has unique needs and problems, an evaluation strategy is usually tailored to these needs. In evaluating a plan, several aspects should be considered:

- Assessment of the quality of care
- Quantification of the accessibility and availability of resources
- Monitoring of the continuity of care
- Measurement of the effectiveness of the care provided
- Evaluation of the acceptability of care provided.

It is helpful to quantify past experience from which comparisons can be made. For example, what existing cost-management programs are in place, and how effective are they? What are the demographic characteristics of the population? What needs improvement?

Each organization should understand the gaps in its benefits package. It is important to stress that isolated or piecemeal approaches to cost containment and plan redesign should be avoided. After all, short-term savings will be illusory if they lead to greater long-term costs. Moreover, tinkering with the present system can be counterproductive *if* appropriate safeguards are not enforced. Evaluation is a prerequisite for any change.

Evaluation is a dynamic process that is bounded by formal application to specific problems. Evaluation should be able to identify the weakness in the benefit plan. Are your prescription drug costs skyrocketing? Is one benefit being overutilized inappropriately? Programs that cost more than they save, divert costs from one category to another or put a different label on an old problem must be assessed. At the root of the problem is the overuse of services and inappropriate use of expensive technology.

Before making changes to the benefits package, before selecting a managed care plan, an employer must know what services and benefits are needed, why they are needed and how much they will cost. As such, it would be wise to start by evaluating the present plan. How much is spent for health care? What has been the plan's experience over five years, for example? What types of services are utilized? What are the high-cost areas? How much is each benefit costing the organization? Are longer-than-expected lengths of stay for specific procedures evident? Are there inappropriate inpatient admissions? What areas would be the most responsive (in both the short term and the long term) to cost-containment efforts and plan redesign? High-cost areas must be identified. Well-designed utilization reports can be used to identify areas that are in need of redesign.

In evaluating the plan, an employer should ask certain basic questions, such as the following:

- Who is covered under the plan? What is the age/sex ratio?
- What has been the cost experience for specific benefits (e.g., hospitalization, drugs, ancillary tests)?
- Does the present plan encourage costly in-hospital stays as opposed to less expensive outpatient treatment?
- What cost-containment programs are currently in effect? How effective have they been?

As a followup to the in-house evaluation, it might be a good idea to compare your results with that of a similar company or trust fund. The Chamber of Commerce of the United States, for example, issues an annual survey of employee benefits; data are analyzed by specific industry and provide an excellent summary of costs and benefits for each industry.

Identification of any problems, or potential problems, should be apparent if a good evaluation of the existing plan is conducted. In many instances, solutions will be self-evident. At this point, it would be beneficial to assess your organization's philosophy that governs employee benefits. What type of aggressive cost-management programs should be implemented? Should you consider self-insurance? What type of managed care program should be considered? Is the present benefit plan meeting the needs and wants of your workforce?

The answers to these questions often determine the nature and scope of cost-containment/cost-management programs. But, before any changes are made, it would be prudent to survey the workforce to ascertain the type of benefits they would like. Surveys can be well worth the time and effort; they can provide useful information for assessing attitudes and can afford employees an opportunity to become more involved in benefits planning. If the package is being utilized inappropriately, neither the employer nor the employee is being well served.

Evaluation is not limited to the large employers. Small and midsize employers should begin using medical claims data to help understand and control their health care costs. Without this information, companies will find it difficult to pinpoint the source of health care cost inflation. A quick look at available data will give you a start on getting the best rate of return on your health care dollars. Key factors to take into consideration include the demographics of the group, the severity of case mix, the excess in utilization, and the cost and charges in the price of services. In particular,

- List the number of admits, days and cost per diem analyzed by diagnosis and type of service.
- Break down data into utilization and unit price to see what factors are driving total costs.
- Assess inpatient versus ambulatory costs to determine where cost savings can be realized.
- List provider charges by type of service and procedure.
- Analyze provider charge against prevailing charges.
- Assess utilization of mental health benefits and calculate costs associated with this care.
- Assess the type of services being used in order to institute preventive health care measures. Are lifestyle-related conditions hurting your bottom line?

Can you state that your utilization management program is effective? Cost trends will help in the decision making regarding changes in benefit plans. The data have to be analyzed to assess cost levels, the direction of the trends and how quickly costs are rising. Remember, however, if improperly analyzed, results can be very misleading and potentially costly to the organization. If the data are not readily available in-house, do not hesitate to request reports from your insurance carrier, third party administrator or benefits consultant.

As the demand for data grows, new means of generating information are proliferating. California's Healthcare Data Information Corporation, set up initially by Pacific Bell to handle claims, has shifted to support clinical data for outcomes analysis. Some of the biggest employers in the state's health industry are part of it. HEDIS 2.0, discussed previously, permits the sharing of data among many employers. In addition, there are numerous proprietary computer programs to help employers generate their own data for analysis. Whatever route one takes, the message is the same: Know where your health care dollars are going, know how effective your benefits package is, and know how you can modify your benefits package to maximize your health care dollars and maintain high quality. Better information systems are being created that can lead to cost savings. Evaluation is the key to your success.

Education and Communication

Hours of planning and expenditure of dollars revising a benefits program do not ensure a smooth working, well-understood benefit plan. Education and communication can. One of the most important aspects of employee benefits planning is to get the message across to all employees regardless of title or rank. The best health plan in the world will not succeed if employees do not understand or are not aware of the provisions in it, especially any changes that have been made. Wrong choices could be made leading to employee dissatisfaction, resentment and potentially higher costs. An education/communication plan is essential. In fact, an education and communication strategy is probably the single most important factor influencing both program utilization and employee acceptance.

In general, employees often look upon changes in their benefits with suspicion. Distrust and misunderstanding could unravel the best conceived plan. Merely updating a benefits booklet will not educate employees about the changes in the plan because most do not read these booklets in the first place. Most people do not read pages filled with words. Be sure that:

- Workers are aware of the problem. Let them know how much health care costs.
- Explanations should be given to employees as to how the organization is containing costs.
- Incentives should be provided to encourage employees to become more cost-conscious consumers.
- A communications program must be implemented over a long period of time. Vary the way your message is delivered.
- All levels of personnel must be included in cost-containment efforts.

The purpose of benefits communication is to explain in clear, simple terms what the employees can expect from the plan. The technical information must be translated into uncomplicated language. What are the options? Eligibility requirements? How much will it cost in terms of deductibles and coinsurance? What requirements must be met? What are the penalties if a managed care plan is not elected? Monitor utilization and satisfaction with the plan. Listen to your employees; you can avoid a great deal of trouble later on by doing so!

A strategy should be developed to clearly identify the goals and objectives of the benefit plan. Mixed or confusing messages about the plan should be avoided. Use of newsletters, special benefits information letters, and pamphlets or brochures explaining benefit changes are often good ways to communicate plan changes. Make your print material eye-catching and easy to read. Use bold typeface to highlight key points. Cartoons or animated characters are a good way to get and hold the reader's attention. However, when explaining numbers or dollar figures, do not be humorous—be clear and precise.

While print material is important to disseminate, it is also very important to provide a forum for employee exchange. Be sure to encourage, indeed welcome, employee input and suggestions. Face-to-face sessions permit employees to ask questions and to have points clarified. As more companies adopt flexible benefit or cafeteria plans and defined contribution plans, the need for personalized communications is paramount. Personal communication is a necessity, not an option.

Audiovisual presentations are an excellent means of getting points across. In this high-tech age, many companies have designed an online information service to assist employees to access both general and individualized information about their benefits any time. If such a computer system is implemented, however, it is imperative that it be user-friendly regardless of the level of computer literacy of the user. The table reviews the advantages and disadvantages of various communication methods.

In summary, education and communication are key ingredients for successful cost-management programs. Be sure that:

- Employees are aware of where their health and welfare dollars are going. Let them know how much their benefits cost.
- Explain clearly how you are working to better manage these costs and how savings will benefit all.
- Educate and communicate, utilizing different means and over a sustained period of time. Education and communication are not a one-shot event.
- Be sure both labor and management are supportive of cost-containment efforts.

Is There a Payoff?

In this era of cost management, it is imperative that each organization assess and evaluate its own benefit plan. Evaluation can play a very important role in identifying areas of potential cost overruns. A little bit of savings here and a little bit of savings there can add up to an impressive figure. But, one needs to know where to look before savings can be realized. Of course, cost savings achieved by one company do not imply that another company will have the same results. Individual employer needs will dictate the scope and direction of changes to the benefits package.

Case studies provide examples of what some employers have done to manage their health care costs:

- * Company X, a multistate health and life insurance company serving over 225,000 covered lives, did an in-house analysis of its claims and discovered numerous improper billing patterns

TABLE

Key Advantages and Disadvantages of Selected Communications Media

1. PRINT

Pros:
—Easiest to develop and control
—Most economical
—Allows for detailed coverage
of complex information
—Several types of print media can be used
for maximum exposure of your message.
—Provides permanent reference for employees

Cons:
—Impersonal, mass produced
—Doesn't usually allow for feedback
—If not perfectly drafted, easy to
misunderstand
—Less impact on changing behavior
or attitudes
—Distribution may be problematic.

2. GROUP MEETINGS

Pros:
—Allow for ultimate flexibility in responding
to specific employee questions/concerns
—Provide a forum for feedback
—Demonstrate employer-union commitment
and openness

Cons:
—Costly
—Difficult to control consistency
—Logistical requirements time-consuming and
labor-intensive
—Require employees to take time away
from work
—Rely on employee memory

3. AUDIOVISUALS (videos, slideshows, etc.)

Pros:
—Familiar mode of taking in information
—Dramatic and visual: leave strong impression
—Easy to understand
—Require clear messages and
identification of key points

Cons:
—Production can be costly and difficult.
—Benefit changes can quickly make an
expensive presentation obsolete.
—Less suitable for complex materials

4. TELEPHONE HOT LINES

Pros:
—Personal
—Flexible, easy to use
—Ideal for dealing with complex issues

Cons:
—Costly
—Labor-intensive
—Must be carefully structured to meet peaks
and valleys in demands for information
—Dependent on telephone company's
implementation schedule

5. COMPUTERS

Pros:
—Allow for detailed and instantaneous
access to information
—Provide for constant updating

Cons:
—Not always easy to use
—Costly
—Not practical unless all employee locations
have access

Source: V. James Gutowski, Barbara W. Sessions and Claude L. Kordus, "Communicating Employee Benefit
Plans," in *Employee Benefits Today: Concepts and Methods,* ed. Claude L. Kordus (Brookfield, WI:
International Foundation of Employee Benefit Plans, 1989), p. 323.

of providers. They purchased a software product designed to detect unbundled claims. Within a short period of time, Company X was saving $40,000 per week in unbundled claims savings. Now they can identify inappropriate claims, deny payments and advise the provider of service accordingly.

* A large investor-owned utility with 55,000 covered lives watched helplessly while its health care costs soared from $21 million to $82 million in less than a decade. The utility realized that aggressive action had to be taken in order to remain solvent. The company implemented incentives to encourage efficient use of health care services, managed utilization of substance abuse services and high-cost health care more aggressively, and established financial incentives to reward employees for appropriate use of services. Within three years, health care costs were $66 million below where they would have been had changes not been implemented. The utility realized that by managing rather than administering their health care benefits, a sizable payoff was realized. Quality did not suffer and a more appropriate use of health care services was evident. Again, evaluation and excellent communication measures helped the utility achieve its goal. The utility has expanded its mission to adopt outcomes measures to further refine its delivery of cost-efficient health care for its employees and dependents.

* Company Y, a Fortune 250 company with 38,000 covered lives, had medical costs that were almost 8% of payroll. Benefit costs were $46 million in 1994 and potentially increasing. An evaluation of where their dollars were being spent showed that 6% of the employees were responsible for 67% of the health care costs. Many services, for example, were being delivered in the emergency room. A plan of action was implemented to include monitoring compliance issues and disease management techniques aimed at employees with chronic diseases. The company incorporated a wellness program as well to address their cost problem. The idea was to encourage employees to embrace healthier lifestyles. The company attributes its savings to these measures.

* A $1.5 billion environmental company with 3,600 employees nationwide shifted to managed care in 1994. Information was initially gathered to help select a managed care organization to

help end the "chaos," as the director of benefits and compensation described the benefits program currently in place. Medical costs have since been reduced by $2 million a year and the benefits program has been made more manageable and efficient.

Summary

While there are scores of other success stories, these examples serve to illustrate how important evaluation and communication are. What is also instructive is that cost savings were achieved within a very short period of time. Obviously, continued monitoring is needed to ensure that the program is working as intended. But, the key message here is that hours of planning and thousands of dollars do not ensure a smooth working, well-understood, cost-efficient benefits program. Communication skills do. While plan redesign can do much to make an organization's benefits package more cost-effective, without the cooperation and understanding of the employees, it would be difficult to achieve the objectives. If employees are made to realize that cost-containment activities are in their best interest, then their cooperation most probably would be forthcoming.

CHAPTER 11

Thoughts for the Future

E vents taking place in the health care sector are happening so fast that it is often difficult to keep abreast of all the changes, and often hard to figure out what to do. It is clear, however, that there are major changes dramatically altering the way health care is delivered and financed. The situation makes it difficult for health and welfare managers and human resource personnel to chart a course that will meet the needs and expectations of the employees but not bankrupt the employer.

Anxiety and concern about the affordability of medical care are palpable. Both management and labor are concerned because rising health care costs threaten industry's economic vitality, its ability to complete and to provide jobs. Individuals are concerned because more of the costs are borne directly by them, which often means that their take-home pay and their standard of living are constrained.

Not surprisingly, a 1996 survey of human resource executives found that the majority felt that the toughest challenge they faced is controlling health care and benefit costs. Concerns about costs, access, quality and efficiency have galvanized the population to focus on reforming the system. While some of the issues are more easily addressed, others are more recalcitrant, less responsive to change. That is, we can do much to prevent the high cost of lifestyle-related diseases such as cancers, heart disease, AIDS and substance abuse. We can try to streamline the hugely inefficient administrative structure, which has created a confusing maze of providers and service delivery organizations. But, taming medical inflation and the ballooning costs of retiree health care are less easily accomplished.

An understanding of the issues is imperative for those involved in planning, administering and managing the health care system. This guide was written to help the reader become familiar with the range of cost-management approaches currently available; to help understand the current terminology; and to assist in the navigation of the managed care system, which seems to be the dominant force in health care delivery and financing.

The chronic nature of the health care cost problem has provided the impetus for public and private organizations to undertake cost-containment initiatives. While many of these efforts have not yielded a desired or expected outcome, others did successfully help restrain spending growth. *But,* no one initiative has slowed the overall health care inflation substantially over the long term. In a sense, the past efforts, however well intended and noble, failed to address the root causes of cost inflation. Political factors often did not help matters; politics frequently have served to torpedo constructive action over the years.

Although the politics of health care reform has created gridlock, the notion that the system is in need of restructuring is still with us. It is just that the configuration of the new system is in dispute. At this writing, it is probably fair to characterize the health care system as one in transition. There have been many such transitions in the past, but the present movement is becoming more vertically integrated, more concentrated and much more concerned with the bottom line. Unfortunately, these changes are taking place in lieu of a formal national policy. The system seems at times to be driving itself.

Thanks to the Reagan administration's laissez-faire approach to the health care market, a largely unregulated, freewheeling environment permitted the proliferation of managed care. Private market forces were given the green light to transform the health care system. Competition was encouraged and a not so subtle shift from nonprofit to for profit became evident. Was this shift a positive force? There have been numerous studies regarding the cost savings potential of competition; most indicate that more competition has led to higher, not lower, prices.

While the industry is still undergoing its own transformation (of note, the flurry of mergers and acquisitions and market consolidation), there is a need to be mindful of the effects (both positive and negative) of this new system. The consolidation of managed care organizations has created situations where potential advantages of competitive markets are negated. Situations exist where a few concentrated players control a high proportion of an area's insured population, thus precluding the opportunity for others to get a toehold in that market. Although the managed care industry is a long way from the concentration we see in the auto sector, for example, in some places in the United States the consolidation/transformation is striking. Minneapolis/St. Paul and Southern California, for example, come to mind immediately.

We have witnessed, in less than ten years, a shift from cost containment (watchword of the 1980s) to cost management (buzzword of the early 1990s) to cost optimization (latest sound bite to describe the forces driving the system). Accountability and measured performances are characteristic of the latter. This shift has not come without pain, however, and the current transition period is difficult for providers and consumers alike.

As this guide has tried to illustrate, there remain serious problems in America's health care system. Few would deny that the system is administratively unwieldy, fragmented, inefficient and costly. Over 20¢ on every dollar is spent just to process paperwork, representing $200 billion in 1994 alone! What does it mean when a system in which total spending is expected to exceed $1 trillion is controlled by a few large entities? With only a few sellers, but lots of buyers, who will discipline the system? Who will be the watchdog? Until the system evolves to the next stage, each consumer must demand accountability. Fortunately, employers are becoming more discerning purchasers of care.

Managed care has brought new dimensions to the system by transforming the way health care is delivered and financed. These changes represent an opportunity as well as a threat: opportunity to reform the delivery and financing systems, and threat that quality of care, research and a pool of well-trained physicians will be sacrificed to short-term profits. Choosing a doctor or hospital is not like selecting a new car or a refrigerator. Dr. Arnold Relman, former editor of the *New England Journal of Medicine,* wrote in 1987:

> In whatever kind of organizational setting physicians practice these days, they must above all be more vigilant than ever to insure that patients' interests are protected. If patients ever lose their trust in the commitment of the medical profession, they and their physicians will be deprived of an element vital to good care, and the quality of medical services will decline. Physicians have an obligation to preserve their patients' trust. It is an obligation quite different from, and often incompatible with, the relations between sellers and buyers in a commercial market. That is why what is

good, i.e., profitable, for the new health care businesses may not be so good for ethical physicians or for the patients they are sworn to serve.

His words still ring true a decade later. We all must be mindful that marketplace issues of cost, efficiency, networking, strategic partnering and enrolling new members do not overshadow the primary concerns of what caregivers are all about and whom they serve.

The problem, however, is how to assess the effectiveness of managed care. The multitude of variables make it difficult to understand how the health care marketplace is likely to function. The decrease in health care spending noted in the mid-1990s may be a temporary lull or may reflect the first sign of a restructuring spurred by managed competition. It is much too early to draw conclusions. Part of the problem is that cost studies have not isolated savings due to managed care mechanisms from savings due to other factors. Without proper adjustments for spending levels, savings due to other changes affecting the local and national health care markets may be credited inappropriately to managed care. If not taken into account, confounding factors such as selection biases, benefit differences, and measurement of quality and cost factors may create a distorted picture of the success of managed care.

Fortunately, employers realize that accurate assessment of the effect of managed care requires data about costs as well as outcomes (including quality of care and patient satisfaction). Employers have demanded that quality must not be the sacrificial lamb in this business. Outcomes research, quality assurance and cost analyses have become important components. Understanding the benefits and risks of treatments and knowing which treatments result in improved outcomes for patients under different circumstances are crucial to ensuring quality. The key to a managed care organization's survival will be documentation of cost-effectiveness *and* quality accountability.

Research in the health sector is needed more than ever. Without it, we would not be able to understand what works and what doesn't work. Further, research is needed to identify information most likely to assist consumers and employers in choosing health plans and to aid in decision making regarding health options. Managed care organizations are trying to show that each can do a better job by ensuring higher quality and better outcomes while using fewer resources—a contradiction of sorts perhaps, but a concept that is driving the industry. It is up to the purchaser, the employer, the trust fund, the individual, to be as informed as possible. Do your homework first; know what your needs are and what options would be most appropriate.

Although there are basic responses to containment of health care costs, differing circumstances and philosophies often will dictate which programs or options will have the best chance of succeeding. However, many different factors contributed to the present situation, and there are no simple solutions, no magic bullets.

The premise maintained herein is that a cost-conscious consumer must become a consumer manager who identifies and purchases quality health care with the same skill and perception employed in purchasing other goods and services. One of the central messages of this volume is that there are options that have the potential of containing costs, thus helping the organization get the most for its benefit dollars. Some of the strategies and initiatives discussed in the preceding chapters can be implemented unilaterally; others may require the involvement of the insurance carrier, managed care organization, hospitals and physicians.

Of central importance is the need to plan. *Planning,* most simply defined, is the process of thinking about the future and taking the necessary steps to address the problems. In particular:

- Identify high-cost areas and eliminate inappropriate and unnecessary services, which should not be too hard to identify if one undertakes an analysis of where the costs are being spent, on whom and for what.
- Identify needs and agree on a strategy.
- Communicate goals and objectives clearly.
- Monitor and evaluate the programs to ensure that the goals are being met.

What every employer should understand, however, is that what may work for others may not work for you. Assessment and evaluation of your situation are imperative in order to achieve the most efficient use of your scarce resources.

The strategies discussed in the guide should provide information for thought and prudent action. Additionally, there are scores of seminars, conferences, newsletters and consultants eager to help you navigate the shark-infested waters. Although the employer makes the decision about the type of health care benefit, it is the employee who should have input; employees are an essential component in any health care plan redesign. What type of benefits would they like? What are their needs? What would they like to see added or deleted from the plan? What do they think about the information they presently receive? What kinds of information do they want to help them select a plan? Surveys of employee attitudes can be well worth the time and effort. They can provide useful information for assessing attitudes and they afford employees an opportunity to become more involved in benefits planning and design. Misdirected cost containment will certainly generate controversy and ill will while falling short of achieving its objectives.

The preceding chapters have highlighted most, but by no means all, of the types of cost-management programs that should be considered. Efforts must be flexible in that strategies should be modified or eliminated if they are not working. Logically, not all cost-containment programs will be acceptable or appropriate. Options should be left open. It must be realized that cost management is a long-term commitment and it may take years to realize savings from some programs.

Indeed, it may take years to determine whether the "reforms" taking place can reduce costs or whether additional mechanisms or additional transformations of the delivery system (such as global budgeting, rate setting or expenditure limits) will be needed. There are many issues which must be addressed before we can celebrate. Just as past efforts at containment failed to control health care costs and medical inflation, the short-term "savings" and "success" of managed care may well fail to address the basic underlying factors that are driving the system.

In summary, cost management is still a necessary component of any health benefits plan. If an organization adopts a do-nothing attitude and does not look carefully and critically at its benefit package, the organization and its employees will be spending hard earned dollars unnecessarily. Clearly, no one can afford to do that any longer. Escalating health care costs affect providers and consumers alike, and all of us must continue to better manage the resources at hand lest we be crushed by the system's inherent inefficiencies.

Glossary of Selected Terms

A **ACCESS:** The ability to obtain needed health services. Measures of access include the location of the health facility, hours of operation, patient travel time/distance to health facility and availability of health services.

ACCOUNTABILITY: An obligation to periodically disclose appropriate information in adequate detail and consistent form to all contractually involved parties.

ACCREDITATION: Formal recognition by an agency or organization which evaluates an institution or organization as meeting certain predetermined standards.

ACCRUAL OF BENEFITS: In the case of a defined benefit pension plan, the process of accumulating pension credits for years of credited service, expressed in the form of an annual benefit to begin payment at normal retirement age. In the case of a defined contribution plan, the process of accumulating funds in the individual employee's pension account.

ACCRUED BENEFIT: For any retirement plan which is not a defined benefit pension plan, a participant's accrued benefit is the balance in his or her plan account, whether vested or not. In the case of a defined benefit pension plan, a participant's accrued benefit is his or her benefit as determined under the terms of the plan expressed in the form of an annual benefit commencing at normal retirement age.

ACUTE CARE: Conditions that are short term or episodic in nature.

ADMINISTRATIVE SERVICES ONLY (ASO): A type of employee benefit plan that is administered by an insurance company or third party administrator and in which the client is totally at risk for claims.

ADMISSION CERTIFICATION: A form of utilization review in which assessment is made of the necessity of a patient's admission to a hospital or other inpatient institution.

ADULT DAY CARE: The provision during the day, on a regular basis, of a range of services that may include health, medical, psychological, social, nutritional and educational services that allow a person to function in the home.

ADVANCE FUNDING: An approach to funding retirement benefits whereby the employer sets aside monies for each employee or for the group of active employees as a whole on some systematic basis during their working years.

ADVERSE SELECTION: A person with an impaired health status or with expected medical care needs applies for insurance coverage financially favorable to himself or herself and detrimental to the insurance company.

AFFILIATION OF HEALTH PROVIDERS: A relationship between an organization operating a project and another health organization under which the latter provides services to the former.

AFTERCARE: Continued care provided after a health treatment.

ALLIED HEALTH PROFESSIONALS: Trained and licensed health care professionals other than physicians, dentists, optometrists, chiropractors, podiatrists and nurses. Examples include physical therapists, pharmacists, medical social workers and home health aides.

ALLOCATED BENEFITS: Benefits for which the maximum amount payable for specific services is itemized in the contract.

ALLOCATED FUNDING INSTRUMENT: A funding instrument by which contributions are assigned to provide benefits for specific employees.

ALLOCATION: The distribution of the employer's contribution to the account of each participant.

ALLOWED COSTS: Charges for services rendered or supplies furnished by a health provider which would qualify as covered expenses and for which the program pays in whole or in part.

ALL-PAYERS SYSTEM: Used in reference to hospital rate setting programs. Subjects to the same rules all third party payers who are reimbursing hospitals for services.

ALTERNATIVE DELIVERY SYSTEM: See Health Maintenance Organization (HMO).

AMBULATORY CARE: Health services rendered in an outpatient facility.

AMBULATORY CARE BENEFITS: Benefits for health care services received as an outpatient.

AMBULATORY DELIVERY SYSTEM: A health care system in which care is provided on an outpatient basis.

ANCILLARY SERVICES: Services exclusive of hospital room and board; include radiography and laboratory tests.

APPROVED PLAN: A pension, deferred profit-sharing or stock bonus plan that meets the requirements of the Internal Revenue Code and the applicable regulations. Such approval qualifies the plan for favorable tax treatment.

ASSIGNMENT OF BENEFITS: The signed transfer of certain benefits by the insured to a third party.

AVERAGE LENGTH OF STAY: The average number of patient days of service rendered to each inpatient during a given period.

BARGAINING CONTRACT: A contract under which both (or all) parties set the terms and conditions of the contract.

BASELINE: Refers to data collection and analysis at a given point in time against which comparisons can be made.

BASIC MEDICAL BENEFITS: Include benefits for hospital, surgical, medical and other miscellaneous employee benefits, excluding major medical insurance.

BENEFICIARY: A person designated by a participant or by the terms of an employee benefit plan who is or may become entitled to a benefit thereunder.

BENEFIT: Rights of the participant to either cash or services after meeting the eligibility requirements of the pension or other benefit plans.

BENEFIT BOOKLET: Booklet for employees that contains explanation of benefits and related provisions of the health plan. See also Summary Plan Description.

BOARD CERTIFICATION: Physicians who have passed an examination given by a medical specialty board and have been certified by that board as specialists in the subject in question.

CAFETERIA PLAN: See Flexible Benefit Plan/Flexible Compensation.

CAPITATION: A fixed predetermined amount paid to a provider for each person served, without regard to the number of services provided to each person in a set period of time. It is the characteristic payment in managed care organizations.

CARVE-OUT: An approach to supplement Medicare in which medical expenses for eligible persons under Medicare are provided on the same basis as for active employees, except for a reduction by Medicare benefits.

CASE MANAGEMENT: Monitoring, planning and coordinating treatment rendered to those with conditions requiring high-cost or extensive services. It is intended to ensure an appropriate and cost-effective course of treatment.

CASE MIX: The classifications or categories of patients treated by a hospital.

CERTIFICATE OF NEED: A certificate issued by a governmental body to an individual or organization proposing to construct or modify a health facility, acquire new medical equipment or offer a new health service. It is intended to control expansion of facilities and services by preventing their excessive or duplicative development.

CERTIFICATION: The process by which a governmental or nongovernmental agency evaluates and recognizes a person who meets predetermined standards. Certification is applied to individuals; accreditation to institutions.

CERTIFIED LENGTH OF STAY: The period of time approved as necessary and appropriate for a patient to receive inpatient care in a hospital.

CHARGES: The dollar amount a hospital assesses on an itemized bill.

CLAIM: An itemized statement of services provided by a health care provider for a given patient, usually for one episode of care or set of services. The claim is submitted to a health benefits plan for payment.

CLAIMS PROCEDURE: Each plan is required to provide a claims procedure which must be explained to plan participants and beneficiaries. The denial of a claim made under the claims procedure must be in writing with an explanation of the reasons for the denial.

CLAIMS REVIEW: Examination of a claim submitted for payment or predetermination of benefits; may include determination of eligibility, coverage of service and plan liability as part of a quality review.

CLASS RATING: The price per unit of insurance is computed for all applicants with a given set of characteristics. It is an approach to rate making.

CLINICAL OUTCOMES: Health status changes or effects that individual patients experience resulting from the delivery of health care usually measured in terms of morbidity, mortality, functional ability and satisfaction with care.

CLINICAL OUTLIERS: Cases that cannot adequately be assigned to an appropriate diagnostic related group because of unique combinations of diagnoses.

CLOSED PANEL: A set list of providers who provide services only at specified facilities.

COALITIONS: Joint collaboration of health care providers, purchasers of care, industry, consumers, labor or insurers in an attempt to deal with health care costs, issues and problems.

COINSURANCE: A policy provision by which both the insured and the insurer share in a specified ratio (usually 80%/20%) of health care expenses.

COLLECTIVE BARGAINING: The process of good faith negotiation between employer and employee representatives concerning issues of mutual interest.

COLLECTIVE BARGAINING AGREEMENT OR CONTRACT: A formal agreement over wages, hours and conditions of employment entered into between an employer or group of employers and one or more unions representing employees.

COLLECTIVELY BARGAINED PLAN: A plan maintained pursuant to an agreement that the secretary of labor finds to be a collective bargaining agreement between employee representatives and one or more employers.

COMBINATION METHODS IN HEALTH CARE: The combination of various types of plans such as self-funded plans for basic coverage and insured plans for supplemental major medical coverage.

COMBINATION PLANS: An agreement under which two funding media are used, with a portion of the contributions placed in a trust fund and the balance paid to an insurance company as contributions under a group annuity contract or as premium on individual life insurance or annuity contracts.

COMBINED PLAN: Most often a Blue Cross-major medical combination.

COMMUNITY MENTAL HEALTH CENTER: Facility or facilities licensed by the state and funded by the federal government to provide mental health services in a designated catchment area.

COMORBIDITY: Diseases that coexist in addition to the index condition.

COMPARISON GROUP: Any group of people to which the index group is compared. Usually synonymous with control group.

COMPENSATION: The amount of wages, salary or earned income an individual receives from services rendered as a result of employment or self-employment.

COMPREHENSIVE MEDICAL CARE: A complete package of health care services and benefits.

COMPREHENSIVE MEDICAL PLAN: A plan that combines basic and major medical coverage in a single plan.

CONCURRENT REVIEW: The process by which hospital admissions are certified for appropriateness and by which continued stays are verified for medical necessity and level of care.

CONTINUED STAY REVIEW: Similar to concurrent review. Also sometimes called recertification.

CONTINUITY OF CARE: The result of a planned treatment program designed to provide the individual patient with the total range of needed services under continuing responsible direction.

CONTRIBUTION: A payment made into a fund by the fund sponsor.

CONTRIBUTION LIMITS: The maximum dollar limit on annual additions (employer contributions, certain employee contributions and forfeitures) for an employee under defined contribution plans of an employer.

CONTRIBUTORY PLAN: A benefit plan under which employees bear part of the cost.

COORDINATION OF BENEFITS (COB): A group health insurance policy provision designed to eliminate duplicate payments and provide the sequence in which coverage will apply when a person is insured under two contracts.

COPAYMENTS: Payments made by consumers (e.g., deductibles and coinsurance) to discourage inappropriate utilization and to help finance health benefit plans.

COST/BENEFIT ANALYSIS: Comparison of the costs with the benefits through elimination of other direct and indirect costs.

COST CONTAINMENT: Activities aimed at holding down the cost of medical care or reducing its rate of increase.

COST REIMBURSEMENT: A method of provider reimbursement based on actual costs incurred.

COST SHARING: Arrangements whereby consumers pay a portion of the cost of health services, sharing costs with employers. Deductibles, co-insurance and payroll deductions are forms of cost sharing.

COST SHIFTING: The burden of health care costs borne by one party or market segment are shifted to another.

COVERAGE: Benefits available to eligible individuals under an employee benefit program.

D **DAMAGES:** The amount claimed or allowed as compensation for injuries sustained through wrongful acts or the negligence of another.

DATABASE: A collection of data stored in computer files

DEDUCTIBLE: The amount of out-of-pocket expenses that must be paid for health services by the insured before becoming payable by the carrier.

DEFERRED COMPENSATION: Arrangements by which compensation to employees for past or current services is postponed until some future date.

DEFERRED COMPENSATION PLAN: Any plan where employees can accumulate money on a tax-deferred basis. It can be combined with other plans such as profit-sharing plans.

DEFINED BENEFIT PLAN: Any plan that is not an individual account plan. There is a definite formula by which the employee's benefits will be measured. The employer's contributions are determined actuarially.

DEFINED CONTRIBUTION PLAN: Any plan which provides for an individual account for each participant and for benefits based on the amount contributed to the participant's account plus any income, expenses, gains, and losses, and forfeitures of accounts of other participants which may be allocated to the participant's account.

DEMAND: The amount of a given health service sought by consumers in response to their perceived need for that service.

DENTAL BENEFIT PLAN: An organized method of financing or providing dental care.

DEPENDENTS: Generally refers to the spouse and children of a covered individual, as defined in a contract.

DIAGNOSTIC RELATED GROUP (DRG): The claims reimbursement system in which payment is based on an episode of care.

DISABILITY: A condition that renders an insured incapable of performing one or more duties of his or her regular occupation.

DISABILITY BENEFIT: Periodic payments payable to participants who are totally or permanently disabled as a result of an injury, illness or disease.

DISABILITY INCOME INSURANCE: A form of health insurance that provides periodic payments to replace income when the insured is unable to work as a result of illness, injury or disease.

DISABILITY RETIREMENT: A termination of employment generally involving the payment of a retirement allowance, as a result of an accident or sickness occurring before a participant is eligible for normal retirement.

DISBURSED SELF-FUNDED PLAN: A type of self-insured or self-funded plan in which employees' claims are paid directly out of the company's cash flow as part of the expense of doing business. Claims settlements are tax deductible when they are paid, not when they are incurred. The company sets aside no reserves and pays no premiums or expense load to an insurer; most buy stop-loss insurance.

DISCHARGE PLANNING: A centralized, coordinated program developed by a hospital to ensure that each patient has a planned program for needed continuing or followup care.

DISEASE MANAGEMENT: An information-based process involving the continuous improvement of value in all aspects of care (prevention, treatment, management). Goals are to affect the outcome of the disease and the long-term cost.

DISEASE PREVENTION: A method of protecting as many people as possible from the consequences of a particular disease or environmental hazard.

DRG RATE: A fixed dollar amount based on averaging of all patients in that DRG in the base year, adjusted for inflation, economic factors and bad debts.

DUAL CHOICE: An option offered individuals in a group to choose between two or more health plans for prepaying medical care.

DUAL OPTION: Refers to federal legislation that requires employers to give their employees the option to enroll in a local HMO rather than in conventional employer-sponsored health program.

DUPLICATION OF BENEFITS: Overlapping or identical coverage of an insured person under two or more health plans. Synonymous with multiple coverage.

EARLY RETIREMENT: Termination of employment involving the payment of a retirement allowance before a participant is eligible for normal retirement.

EARLY RETIREMENT AGE: An age, established by the terms of an employee pension benefit plan, which is earlier than normal retirement age, at which a participant may receive benefits under the plan.

EFFECTIVENESS: The degree to which action(s) achieve the intended health result under normal or usual circumstances.

EFFICACY: Whether an intervention works under controlled conditions.

ELECTIVE SURGERY: An operation or surgical procedure for a condition that is not considered an emergency or life threatening.

ELIGIBLE EMPLOYEES: Those members of a group who have met the eligibility requirements under a group life, health insurance or pension plan.

ELIGIBLE EMPLOYER: Qualified as a tax-exempt organization under Section 101(6) or Section 501(c)(3) of the Internal Revenue Code.

ELIGIBLE EXPENSES: Medical expenses for which a health insurance policy will provide benefits.

ELIGIBILITY DATE: The date an individual and/or dependents become eligible for benefits under an employee benefit plan.

ELIGIBILITY REQUIREMENTS: Conditions that an employee must satisfy to participate in a plan.

EMPLOYEE ASSISTANCE PLAN (EAP): A plan designed to help employees whose job performance is being adversely affected by personal problems.

EMPLOYEE BENEFIT PLAN: A plan established or maintained by an employer or employee organization, or both. The purpose is to provide employees with a certain benefit such as pension, profit sharing, stock bonus, thrift, medical, accident or disability benefits.

EMPLOYEE BENEFIT TRUST: A trust established to hold the assets of an employee benefit plan.

EMPLOYEE HEALTH EDUCATION: A program to encourage good health habits; often referred to as health promotion programs.

EMPLOYEE RETIREMENT INCOME SECURITY ACT OF 1974 (ERISA): Established an insurance program designed to guarantee workers receipt of pension benefits if their defined benefit pension plan should terminate. ERISA regulates the majority of private pension and welfare group benefit plans in the United States.

EMPLOYEE WELFARE BENEFIT PLAN: A plan maintained for the purpose of providing benefits, other than pension benefits, to its participants or their beneficiaries through the purchase of insurance or otherwise.

ENROLLED GROUP: Persons with the same employer or with membership in an organization in common who are enrolled in a health plan.

ENROLLEE: Any person eligible as either a subscriber or a dependent in accordance with an employee benefit plan.

ENROLLMENT: The process by which an individual and/or dependent becomes a subscriber to health plan coverage.

EVALUATION: An examination of and judgment about the quality of services or programs based on predetermined criteria/standards.

EXCLUSIONS OR EXCEPTIONS: Specific conditions or circumstances listed in the policy or employee benefit plan for which the policy or plan will not provide benefit payments.

EXCLUSIVE PROVIDER ORGANIZATION/ARRANGEMENT: An indemnity or service plan that provides benefits or levels of benefits only if care is rendered by institutional and professional providers within a specified network.

EXPERIENCE-RATED PREMIUM: A premium based on the anticipated claims experience of, or utilization of service by, a contract group according to its age, sex and any other attributes expected to affect its health service utilization.

EXPERIENCE RATING: The process of determining the premium rate for a group risk, wholly or partially on the basis of that group's experience.

EXPLANATION OF BENEFITS: A description of benefits received and services for which the health care provider has requested payment.

EXTENDED BENEFITS: A term that can mean comprehensive benefits provided in excess of basic health care plans. It can also refer to extension of benefits for limited periods after termination of plan coverage.

EXTENDED CARE FACILITY: A health care facility offering skilled nursing care, rehabilitation and convalescent services.

EXTERNAL EVALUATION: An evaluation performed by a person or agency not under the direct control of the individual, group or organization being evaluated.

F **FEE FOR SERVICE:** The method of billing for health services under which a health provider charges separately for each service rendered as contrasted with capitation and fee schedules.

FEE SCHEDULE: A listing of fees or allowances for specified medical procedures which usually represents the maximum amounts the program will pay for specified procedures.

FIRST DOLLAR COVERAGE: A benefit plan which provides reimbursement for incurred health care costs from the first dollar, with no deductible.

FLEXIBLE BENEFIT PLAN/FLEXIBLE COMPENSATION: A benefit program that offers employees a choice between permissible taxable benefits and nontaxable health and welfare benefits. The employee determines how his or her benefit dollars are to be allocated for each type of benefit from the total amount promised by the employer.

FLEXIBLE SPENDING ACCOUNTS: Employees are given a choice between taxable cash and nontaxable compensation in the form of payment or reimbursement of eligible, tax-favored welfare benefits. These accounts can be funded through salary reduction, employer contributions or a combination of both.

401(k) PLAN: A defined contribution plan established by an employer. It enables employees to make pretax contributions by salary reduction agreements structured within the format of a cash or deferred plan.

FRINGE BENEFITS: Benefits partially or fully excluded from an employee's gross income and which are not subject to payroll taxes but whose costs are deductible by the employer. Such benefits typically include health, dental and accident benefits; disability benefits; group term life insurance coverage; employee death benefits; and group legal.

FULL VESTING: That form of immediate or deferred vesting under which all accrued benefits of a participant become vested benefits.

GGATEKEEPER: Usually a primary care provider who is responsible for managing medical treatment.

GROSS DOMESTIC PRODUCT: The measure of the economy which includes the market value of goods and services produced.

GROUP PRACTICE: A group of providers engaged in the coordinated practice of medicine.

HEALTH INSURANCE: Protection that provides payment of benefits for covered sickness or injury.

HEALTH MAINTENANCE ORGANIZATION (HMO): A prepaid medical group practice plan that provides a predetermined medical care benefit package. HMOs are both insurers and providers of health care.

HEALTH PROMOTION: Activities related to individual lifestyle to prevent disease, disability and injury.

HEALTH SYSTEM: All of the services, functions and resources in a geographic area, the primary purpose of which is to affect the state of health of the population.

HOME HEALTH AGENCY: An organization providing skilled nursing and other therapeutic services in the patient's home.

HOME HEALTH SERVICES: Items and services provided as needed in patients' homes by a home health agency or by others under arrangements made by a home health agency.

HOSPICE: A health care facility or service providing medical care and support services such as counseling to terminally ill persons.

HOSPITAL BENEFITS: Benefits provided under a policy for hospital charges incurred by an insured person because of an illness or injury.

I **INDEMNITY:** A benefit paid by an insurer for a loss insured under a policy.

INDEMNITY CONTRACT: A contract in which the amount of the benefit is based on the actual amount of financial loss as determined at the time of loss.

INDEMNITY PLAN: The provision of specific cash payment reimbursement for designated covered services. Payments can be made either to enrollees or on assignment directly to health providers. See also Modified Indemnity Plan.

INDIVIDUAL PRACTICE ASSOCIATION (IPA): A type of HMO that consists of a central administrative authority and a panel of physicians and other providers practicing individually or in small groups in the community. Providers are usually reimbursed individually on a fee-for-service or capitation basis.

INDIVIDUAL RETIREMENT ACCOUNT (IRA): A retirement savings program for individuals to which yearly tax-deductible contributions up to a specified limit can be made. The amounts contributed are not taxed until withdrawal, which is not permitted without penalty until age 59½.

INPATIENT: A person who occupies a hospital bed, crib or bassinet while under care or treatment for at least 24 hours.

INSURANCE: A means of providing or purchasing protection against some of the economic consequences of loss.

INSURED: The person to whom or on whose behalf benefits are payable under a policy.

INTEGRATED NETWORKS: Combination or integration of managed care networks into one entity.

INTERMEDIATE CARE FACILITY: An institution licensed under state law to provide, on a regular basis, health care and services to individuals who do not require the degree of care and treatment that a hospital or a skilled nursing facility is designed to provide.

INTERNAL EVALUATION: Evaluation performed by a person or agency that is part of the organization being evaluated.

J **JOINT COMMISSION ON THE ACCREDITATION OF HOSPITALS:** National agency established to periodically inspect hospitals and to grant accreditation in recognition of satisfactory performance.

K **KEOGH PLAN:** A retirement plan for self-employed persons and their employees to which yearly tax-deductible contributions up to a specified limit can be made if the plan meets certain requirements of the IRS.

L **LABOR FORCE:** All persons over age 16 who are employed; does not include persons not looking for work.

LENGTH OF STAY: The expected length of time for which institutionalized patients in a hospital or other health care facility are expected to stay.

LIFE EXPECTANCY: The length of time a person of a given age is expected to live.

LIFETIME DISABILITY BENEFIT: Payment to help replace income lost by an insured person as long as he or she is totally disabled, even for a lifetime.

LONG-TERM CARE: Provision of health, personal and social services to individuals who lack some functional capacity (e.g., chronically ill, elderly, disabled). Care is provided on a long-term basis in institutions or at home.

LONG-TERM DISABILITY INCOME INSURANCE: Insurance issued to an employer group or individual to provide reasonable replacement of a portion of an employee's earned income lost through serious and prolonged illness or injury during the normal work career.

LOSS OF BENEFITS: An employee's right to accrued benefits from personal contribution is not subject to forfeiture under any circumstances.

MAJOR MEDICAL COVERAGE: Type of coverage that usually pays only a portion of the expense for all covered services and specifies a deductible that the insured must first pay. Full reimbursement is often provided once the expenses paid by the individual reach a certain level.

MALPRACTICE: A deviation from professional duty or failure of professional skill or learning that results in death, injury, loss or damage to the patient.

MANAGED CARE: Management of utilization, quality and claims using a variety of current cost-containment methods. The primary goal is to deliver cost-effective care without sacrificing quality or access.

MANDATED BENEFITS: A specific set of benefits required by law to be provided by all insurance carriers and reimbursed under all insurance policies.

MARKET: Sets of all people who have an actual or potential interest in a product or service.

MARKET ANALYSIS: An analytic process associated with planning that is initiated for the purpose of defining and characterizing the market and its needs, wants or preferences.

MARKET AREA: A place or location associated with the actual or potential markets that an organization targets or selects for delivery of one or more products or services.

MARKET SEGMENT: A subset of a larger market.

MEDICAL CASE MANAGEMENT: Coordinated care of high-cost claims and specialized care and services. Most often is used to deal with catastrophic illnesses. The coordinator oversees overall management of care.

MEDICARE SUPPLEMENT POLICY (MEDIGAP POLICY): A voluntary, contributory private insurance plan available to Medicare eligible to cover the costs of physician services and other medical and health services not covered by Medicare.

MINIMUM PREMIUM PLAN: Employer and insurer agree that the employer will be responsible for paying all claims up to an agreed-upon aggregate level, with the insurer responsible for the excess.

MODIFIED INDEMNITY PLAN: Like traditional indemnity plans, modified plans pay providers on a fee-for-service basis, allow patients to have full freedom of choice of providers and require patients/employees to pay a portion of the cost of care through deductibles, coinsurance and contributions. The employer and/or insurer bears the majority of the financial risk. Cost-containment/utilization review controls are used.

MORBIDITY: The condition of being affected by a disease, illness or symptoms.

MORTALITY: Death.

MULTIEMPLOYER PLAN: Plan maintained pursuant to a collective bargaining agreement to which two or more employers contribute. Employer contributions to the plan must be set forth in the labor agreement.

MULTIOPTION PLAN: A plan which offers employees the opportunity to choose the type of health insurance coverage they prefer. Common is the triple option plan consisting of an HMO, a PPO and a modified indemnity plan.

N **NATIONAL HEALTH INSURANCE:** Any system of socialized health insurance benefits, covering all or nearly all citizens, established by federal law, administered by the federal government and supported or subsidized by taxation.

NETWORK: A group of providers that mutually contract with carriers or employers to provide health care services to participants in a specified managed care plan. The contract determines the payment method and rate, utilization controls and target utilization rates by plan participants.

NONCONTRIBUTORY PROVISION: The employer bears the full cost of the benefits for the employees. One hundred percent of eligible employees must be insured.

NONDISABLING INJURY: An injury that may require medical care but does not result in loss of working time or income.

NONQUALIFIED PLAN: A plan that does not meet the requirements of Section 401(a) of the IRS Code and suffers distinct disadvantages from a tax viewpoint.

NOT-FOR-PROFIT THIRD PARTIES: Service corporations or prepayment plans organized under state not-for-profit statutes to provide health care coverage. Blue Cross and Blue Shield plans are examples.

O **OBJECTIVE:** A specific statement that indicates in measurable terms what an organization intends to accomplish and when, in order to progress toward fulfillment of a goal.

OCCUPANCY RATE: The ratio of actual patient days to the maximum patient days as determined by bed capacity during any given period.

OPEN ENROLLMENT: The period during which subscribers in a health benefit program have an opportunity to select an alternate health plan being offered to them.

OUTCOMES MANAGEMENT: The optimization of health outcomes through the continuous development of clinical guidelines and interventions as well as the monitoring and evaluating of data.

OUTCOMES MEASUREMENT: The evaluation of how well a given medical intervention is meeting the health and cost goals of plan sponsors as well as patients.

OUTCOMES RESEARCH: The assessment of effectiveness of a given product, of a disease or of a procedure on health and/or cost outcomes to provide scientific basis for practice guidelines.

OUTLIERS (FOR DRG USE): Not within the norm; i.e., high or low length of stay, clinical outliers.

OUTPATIENT SERVICES: Services provided without a hospital stay.

OVERTREATMENT: Providing more services than are consistent with or justified by diagnosis and treatment plan; synonymous with overutilization.

P

PAID CLAIMS: The dollar value of all claims paid during a plan year.

PARTIAL DISABILITY: An illness or injury which prevents an insured person from performing one or more of the functions of his or her regular job.

PARTIAL HOSPITALIZATION: A therapeutic program that provides less than 24-hour care.

PATIENT CARE EVALUATION STUDY: The process in which an in-depth assessment of the quality and/or nature of the utilization of an aspect of health care services is conducted.

PATIENT DAYS: The accumulated total of the number of patients in a hospital each day; i.e., one patient in one hospital bed for one day.

PAY AS YOU GO: Paying pension benefits as they become due without advance funding.

PEER REVIEW GROUP: Third party reviewers comprised of local physicians who help solve claim disputes and promote fair and ethical practices in the health care industry.

PEER REVIEW ORGANIZATION: A professionally sponsored system for the rendering of professional judgment about quality or appropriateness of health care treatment and related matters.

PER DIEM RATE: Methods of calculation for hospital or health care facility charge.

PHYSICIAN-HOSPITAL ORGANIZATIONS: Alliances between physicians and hospitals to help providers attain market share, improve bargaining power and reduce administrative costs. These entities sell their services to managed care organizations or directly to employers.

PLAN PARTICIPANT: An individual eligible to receive a benefit of any type from an employee benefit plan.

PLAN SPONSOR: The entity sponsoring a benefit plan; i.e., employer, employer organization, joint board of trustees.

PLAN TERMINATION: ERISA requires that all accrued benefits must be fully vested upon termination or partial termination of a plan.

POINT-OF-SERVICE PLAN: Similar to a multioption plan except that employees decide at the time they need health care services whether they will use a managed care provider or an out-of-network provider. These plans combine a high level of employee choice of provider with strong incentives to use managed care alternatives.

PORTABILITY: The provision for retaining pension rights when changing from one employer to another.

PRACTICE GUIDELINES: Systematically developed statements, based on the best scientific evidence, designed to assist practitioners regarding appropriate care for specific clinical circumstances.

PREADMISSION REVIEW: A review and an initial determination by a utilization review committee prior to admission to a hospital of the necessity and appropriateness of the patient's elective admission to a facility level care.

PREADMISSION TESTING: The provision of diagnostic services on an ambulatory basis before an elective hospital admission in order to reduce hospital length of stay.

PREDETERMINATION (PRE-AUTHORIZATION; PRECERTIFICATION): The health provider submits a treatment plan before treatment is initiated.

PREEXISTING CONDITION: A physical and/or mental condition of an insured that existed prior to the issuance of his or her policy.

PREFERRED PROVIDER ORGANIZATION (PPO): A group of hospitals/physicians who contract on a fee-for-service basis with employers, insurance plans or other third party administrators to provide comprehensive medical service.

PREPAID HEALTH PLANS: Health benefit plans that provide a defined set of health services to an enrolled population for a predetermined premium.

PREPAYMENT: A method providing in advance for the cost of predetermined benefits for a population group through regular periodic payments in the form of premiums, dues or contributions.

PRESCRIPTION DRUG PLAN: A plan whereby the beneficiary can obtain prescription drugs without incurring potentially large out-of-pocket expense. The most popular are discount plans, closed panel drug plans, service delivered plans, mail-order plans and maintenance drug options with major medical plans.

PREVAILING FEE: The most commonly charged fee for a service in a given area.

PREVENTIVE CARE: Comprehensive care emphasizing priorities for prevention, early detection and early treatment of conditions, including routine physician examinations, immunizations and well-person care.

PRIMARY CARE: Basic or general health care offered at the time a patient seeks treatment.

PRIMARY CARE NETWORK: A form of alternative delivery system in which health plan enrollees are required to sign up with a primary care practitioner that will handle routine health care needs and serve as gatekeeper. The primary care physician arranges referrals and supervises other care.

PRIOR AUTHORIZATION: The eligibility of a patient to receive certain services and the medical necessity for those services are documented prospectively. Prior authorization may be required for hospital admissions and/or for referral to certain types of ancillary services or to out-of-network providers. Synonymous with preadmission review.

PRO-COMPETITION: The use of competition to identify more efficient and conservative providers and to furnish incentives to participants to choose such providers.

PRODUCTIVITY: The relationship between *output* and *input*, or the amounts of labor, material and capital needed to produce goods and services.

PROSPECTIVE PAYMENT SYSTEM: A payment method in which hospital rates are set prospectively and are based on expected classes and volumes of patients.

PROSPECTIVE RATE SETTING: Financial remuneration of health care providers through a rate established prior to the period to which the rate is to be applied, resulting in the provider being paid the established rate regardless of actual costs.

PROSPECTIVE REVIEW: Requires the granting of authorization for payment before medical care is provided.

PROVIDER: Any health care facility or professional licensed to provide one or more health care services to patients.

PRUDENT BUYER PRINCIPLE: The principle that Medicare should not reimburse a provider for a cost that is not a reasonable cost because it exceeds the amount that a prudent and cost-conscious buyer would be expected to pay.

QUALIFIED PLAN: A plan which the IRS approves as meeting the requirements of Section 401 (a) of the Code. Such plans receive tax advantages.

QUALITY ASSESSMENT: The assessment, measurement or judgment of the quality of health care and the implementation of any necessary changes to either maintain or improve the care rendered.

QUALITY OF CARE: Generally includes the appropriateness and medical necessity of care provided, the appropriateness of the provider who renders care, and the degree to which health care services are delivered in accordance with established professional standards of structure, process and outcome.

QUALITY REVIEW COMMITTEE: A committee to assess and assure quality.

REASONABLE AND CUSTOMARY CHARGE: The prevailing charge made by surgeons of similar expertise for a similar procedure in a particular geographic area.

REHABILITATION: The provision of some long-term disability policies that provides for continuation of benefits and other financial assistance while a totally disabled insured is retraining or attempting to resume productive employment.

RELATIVE VALUE SCALE: A method of determining benefits based on establishing unit values as norms for various medical and surgical procedures, relating the value of each procedure to others by using a conversion factor to arrive at a dollar value for benefits.

RESOURCE-BASED RELATIVE VALUE SCALE (RBRVS): A system of reimbursement for the Medicare program taking into account physician behavior, price and volume of services, and geographic differences in an effort to establish greater control over expenditures.

RETIREMENT, NORMAL AGE: The earliest age at which an employee is normally entitled to retire with full benefits.

RETROSPECTIVE REIMBURSEMENT: A method of payment to a health provider when payment is made after the services are rendered on the basis of costs incurred by the provider.

RISK FACTORS: Conditions that influence a person's health and are capable of provoking ill health, including inherited or biological, environmental, and behavioral risk factors.

RISK POOL: The portion of provider fees or capitation payments that is withheld as financial reserves to cover unanticipated utilization of services in a managed care system.

RISK SHARING: The method by which premiums and costs of medical protection are shared by plan sponsors and participants.

SCHEDULES PLAN: A health plan that provides specific allowances for each type of medical care and treatment.

SCREENING: The assessment of individuals considered to be at risk for specific conditions and/or diseases. Also, the assessment of individuals who do not conform to predetermined quality guidelines and require additional investigation.

SECOND SURGICAL OPINION PROGRAM: Either a voluntary option or a mandatory requirement for patients who have been recommended for elective surgery.

SELECTIVE CONTRACTING: The negotiation by third party payers of a limited number of contracts with health care professionals and facilities in a given service area. Preferential reimbursement practices and/or benefits are then offered to patients seeking care from these providers.

SELF-ADMINISTERED PLAN: A plan administered by the employer or welfare fund without recourse to an intermediate insurance carrier.

SELF-INSURANCE (SELF-FUNDING): A plan collects no premiums and assumes no risk. In a sense, the employer or fund is acting as an insurance company by paying claims with the money ordinarily earmarked for premiums.

SELF-PAY OPTION: An opportunity offered to laid-off workers or those with insufficient hours worked to maintain eligibility for health benefits through the individual's payment of a premium, thus avoiding lapses in coverage.

SENTINEL EFFECT: A positive effect of utilization review that is not readily quantifiable. Providers knowing that they are going to be reviewed would be more likely to make more prudent recommendations than otherwise.

SERVICE AREA: The geographic area from which a particular health care program draws the majority of its users.

SERVICE BENEFIT: An insurance benefit that fully pays the specific hospital or medical care services rendered.

SKILLED NURSING FACILITY: A facility licensed to provide inpatient care of persons requiring skilled nursing services for a chronic disease or convalescence over a prolonged period of time.

SLIDING FEE SCALE: A fee schedule under which the fee charged varies with the patient's ability to pay.

STAFF MODEL HMO: An HMO in which professional providers within a multispecialty group practice are salaried employees of the HMO.

STOP-LOSS INSURANCE: A form of reinsurance that reimburses employers for all or part of their costs above a predetermined threshold amount.

STRATEGIC PLANNING: A systematic process for setting future direction, developing effective strategies, and ensuring that an organization's structure and systems are compatible with long-term survival and success.

SUBROGATION: The right of the employer or insurance company to recoup benefits paid to participants through legal suit if the action causing the disability and subsequent medical expenses was the fault of another individual. Used as a cost-containment measure.

SUMMARY PLAN DESCRIPTION: A requirement of ERISA for a written statement of a plan in an easy-to-read format. Includes eligibility requirements, coverage, employee rights and appeal procedures.

SUPPLEMENTAL BENEFITS: Benefits provided by a pension plan in addition to normal retirement benefits.

SUPPLEMENTAL MEDICAL INSURANCE (also known as Medicare Part B): The voluntary insurance program which provides insurance benefits for physicians and other medical services.

TECHNOLOGY ASSESSMENT: Evaluation of the safety, effectiveness, efficiency and appropriateness of devices, medical and surgical procedures, and pharmaceuticals as promoted for improving a patient's condition or quality of life.

TERTIARY CARE: Specialized care such as select rehabilitation services, highly technical medical procedures, and burn centers.

THIRD PARTY ADMINISTRATOR: Any organization that pays or insures health care expenses on behalf of beneficiaries or recipients who pay premiums for such coverage.

THIRD PARTY PAYER: An insurer who pays for the services provided to a patient.

THIRD PARTY PAYMENT: Payment for health care when the beneficiary is not making payment in whole or in part on his or her own behalf.

TOTAL COMPENSATION: The value of direct pay plus benefit package.

TOTAL DISABILITY: An illness or injury that prevents an insured person from continuously performing every duty pertaining to his or her occupation or from engaging in any other type of work for remuneration.

TRADITIONAL INDEMNITY PLAN: Generally refers to fee-for-service plans in which the patient chooses whichever doctor and hospital he or she wants to use. Employers pay premiums to insurance companies to cover the costs of providing benefits and administering claims. These plans are usually experienced rated.

TRUST FUND PLAN: A plan under which all or some of the benefits are provided through a trust fund.

UNFUNDED DEFERRED COMPENSATION AGREEMENT: A contract between employer and employee to pay certain sums of money at any later date, usually upon retirement, without payment by the employer into any funding agency.

UNION-SPONSORED PLAN: A program of health benefits developed by a union. Funds to finance the benefits are usually paid out of a welfare fund which receives income from employer contributions, employer and union member contributions or union members alone. The union may operate the plan directly or contract for the benefits.

USUAL, REASONABLE AND CUSTOMARY FEES: Reimbursement based on physicians' usual charge for a given procedure, the amount customarily charged for the service by other physicians in the area and the reasonable cost of services for a given patient after medical review of the case.

UTILIZATION MANAGEMENT: The management of cost, quality and outcome. The focus is on medical effectiveness and efficiency. Crucial is the application of clinically valid criteria and guidelines to quantify outcomes.

UTILIZATION REVIEW: The process of reviewing the appropriateness and the quality of care provided to patients to determine whether health care services are appropriate and necessary and provided in the most cost-effective manner. Review may be prospective, concurrent or retrospective.

V **VESTED BENEFIT:** Accrued benefits that have become nonforfeitable under the vesting schedule adopted by the plan.

VISION CARE COVERAGE PLAN: A separate plan covering medical treatment relating to eye conditions.

W **WELFARE PLANS:** Plans that provide medical, surgical or hospital care or benefits in case of sickness, accident, disability, death or unemployment.

WELLNESS (HEALTH PROMOTION) PLANS: Educational and other programs designed to inform individuals about healthy lifestyles and to direct them to programs and facilities that encourage and support these behaviors. Employers may initiate these programs as part of larger efforts to control health care costs, reduce absenteeism and strengthen employee relations.

WORKERS' COMPENSATION: Every state has a system of providing for the cost of medical care and weekly payments to employees who suffer job-related illnesses or injuries, and to dependents of those killed in industry. Absolute liability is imposed on the employer, which is required to pay benefits prescribed by law.

WRAPAROUND PLAN: A major medical plan and a basic surgical/regular medical plan are wrapped around a basic hospital plan and cover all charges other than those provided for by the basic hospital plan.

Y **YEAR OF PARTICIPATION:** The period of service beginning at the earliest date on which an employee is a participant in the plan and which is required to be taken into account for vesting purposes.

Index

A
Abuser, identity of, 106-107
Americans with Disabilities Act of 1990 (ADA),
130-131
see also Workers' compensation
Any willing provider, 59

B
Benefits *see* Employee benefits
Blood pressure screening, *see* Hypertension
programs

C
Communication
need for, 160-162
types of, 162-165

D
Deferred compensation plans, 36
Dental plans, 41-43
Disability, 129-130
see also Workers' compensation